Home Remedies, Poultices, Salves, & Tinctures

First DJK Publishing House edition published 2020.

Cover Art designed by Pintado

Disclaimer: The recipes contained in this publication are 'olde tyme' recipes that were handed down over generations. Every effort was made by the author to ensure accuracy and validity but neither can be assumed by the reader. Additionally, these recipes are not meant as a substitute for, or used to alter, any medical treatment or therapy without your doctor's advice. This is especially true for pregnant and/or nursing mothers. The author and publisher assume no liability for the use, misuse, or effectiveness from any recipe contained herein.

Published in the United States by

DJK Publishing House

KDP ISBN 979-8-600-37348-8

Print and electronic distribution by Kindle Direct Publishing.

Home Remedies, Poultices, Salves, & Tinctures

By: David J. Kershner

Table of Contents

Introduction

This book represents the culmination of many of my own personal pursuits. As an avid gardener, I have long been skeptical of eager 'script writing physicians' and never understood why generations and centuries worth of herbal and plant knowledge was being disregarded and replaced by man-made synthesized chemicals.

I am also an author who enjoys doing the research almost as much as I do writing.

That being said, the concept for *Home Remedies, Poultices, Salves & Tinctures* is something that has been mulled over by me for quite some time. Without getting on too tall of a soapbox, I personally believe that, as a country, we are the most drugged nation on the face of the planet. Newspapers, magazines, radio, television... everywhere you turn, they all contain advertising for the latest and greatest drug. It's to the point now that patients are taking the advice of nebulous online resources and telling the doctor what the ailments is, what to prescribe, the specific dosage, and the number of refills (duration) required.

In the interests of transparency and disclosure, I also write fictional works. It just so happened that the piece I was working on took place several decades after a cataclysmic event where modern medicine no longer existed. As I was working on the piece, given my previously mentioned belief, I found myself asking the same questions repeatedly; 'How am I going to address this issue?' and 'What did we do before all of this?'

Well, back in the day, and to be clear I am generally referring to pre-Industrial Revolution and in some cases as recent as WWII, a lot of the country, and the world for that matter, used home remedies, poultices, salves, and tinctures.

Queue the research!

Many of the recipes contained herein are 'olde tyme' recipes that were handed down over generations so no one knows where or how they originated. However, for the recipes where I thought I located an 'author', either they were non-responsive to repeated requests or they chose to demure and opt for anonymity. In their words, "Many of these recipes have been around for ages... grandma's, grandma's, mother-in-in-law type stuff. It wouldn't be right to take credit."

As with anything, no recipe is perfect. Readers are encouraged to try any of the items in this collection and adjust them accordingly based on a variety of personal factors like allergy concerns, pregnancy, quantity, preference, genetic predisposition, etc.

Finally, please don't take these potential solutions as Gospel. Some of these remedies may not work for you. Make adjustments as necessary then try a different combination of ingredients until you find one that does the job.

Disclaimer: Every effort was made by the author and publisher to ensure accuracy and validity but neither can be assumed by the reader. Additionally, these recipes are not meant as a substitute for, or used to alter, any medical treatment or therapy without your doctor's advice. This is especially true for pregnant and/or nursing mothers. The author and publisher assume no liability for the use, misuse, or effectiveness from any recipe or information contained herein.

Foreword

The concept of alternative medicine began simply as medicine. Many of the things that we look at as real medicine today, have their roots in what we today refer to as tinctures, snake oil, or an alternative. The concept of Tylenol or Motrin began as chewing the bark from a specific tree. Today, we live in a society that insists on pure and clean products that have been manufactured in a sterile room. Similar results would have been found had the product been pulled from nature, boiled, and strained at home then swallowed down the old-fashioned way. The balance today between going to the drug store and talking to your grandparents about how best to deal with certain ailments often times depends on your willingness to try something new to you. Our elders have been using remedies as described in this book for multiple generations before to combat, successfully mind you, the very same issue.

Remember, unsuccessful remedies are rarely recalled other than to say they didn't work. The recipes that do are passed down throughout the years.

Through years of medical training, I learned a vast array of techniques and medicines for the treatment of all manner of illness and infection. However, through fellowship training in holistic and alternative medicine, I learned that there are choices. Like our ancestors, many of the determinations of what works best for you will come from trial and error. It is in publications such as this that help better focus your natural medicinal journey.

Dr. A. E. Notham, D.O.
Family Medicine, Alternative, and Holistic Medicine
Chief of Staff

Chapter 1: Oils

When people visit an herb garden, they touch and sniff the plants. It's almost an involuntary reaction. The reasons behind this could be anything from a connection to the Earth to the enjoyment of the fragrance or the flavors added when cooking. Regardless of the reason, utilizing oils containing these herb and plant matter ingredients allows the person to further that connection to the plant.

That being said, there are two types of oils generally associated with home remedies, poultices, salves, and tinctures. They are essential oils and infused oils. In lay terms:

- Essential oils are oils expressed from plant matter (flower, leaf, stem, and roots)
- Infused oils are oils where the plant matter ingredients are steeped like tea.

Essential Oils

An essential oil is an ingredient used in many salves and soaps. The term 'essential oil' refers more to the inclusion of the ingredients 'essence' than to the required or indispensable nature of the ingredient. The 'essence' of the plant can be loosely defined as the 'fragrant' parts of the plant. The fragrant parts are complex mixtures of naturally occurring chemicals that act as powerful attractants to insects to insure pollination. They can also provide protection by repelling harmful insects. In addition, essential oils are not an 'oil' in the strictest sense of the word. Oils are lipids, or fat. However, essential oils often share oil like qualities in that they have poor solubility in water.

An essential oil can be derived from just about anything. Many indigenous peoples the world over often used, and still use, specific plants, or plant combinations, to generate all manner of remedy. However, modern science being what it is, says that there are some hazards when dealing with the generation of essential oils and with the handling of the finished product.

First, they (modern science) state that essential oils are volatile. However, the caveat to this is that the volatility generally only applies to bulk manufacturing in perfumers and factories. Places where large quantities of the oil are present through either storage or generation. The reason they are considered volatile is because, as opposed to most other oils we deal with on a daily basis, oils like olive, corn, vegetable, safflower, coconut, the essential oils have a lower boiling point and the specific temperature can vary wildly depending on the plant.

The term volatile is also applied to essential oils because they consist of tiny molecules that evaporate when exposed to air, even at normal room temperatures. Rates of evaporation vary among different essential oils too. Be warned though, essential oils will oxidize and lose their therapeutic action when left in the heat or light, so they are best stored in dark glass containers which are also sometimes referred to as 'tincture bottles'.

Rest assured though, there are safety guidelines that have been generally accepted and associated with essential oils. Some of these include:

- External use only
- Pregnant women should exercise extreme caution and use only citrus oils (not in the sun) and lavender oil
  o Other Essential Oils should be used with caution during pregnancy
  o Some citrus oils are phototoxic, meaning they can cause permanent discoloration of the skin when the skin is exposed to the sun
- Less is better
- Keep out of eyes
- Keep out of the reach of children
- Test patch for skin sensitivity

Carrier oils (oils extracted from nuts, seeds, fruits and vegetables) are used to dilute essential oils when applying to the skin. In so doing, it protects the skin from possible irritation by diluting the highly concentrated essential oil.

Making essential oils is done by extracting the natural oils from herbs and/or flowers. As far as extraction is concerned, essential oils can be expressed through various means from all parts of plants. "All parts" means the roots, bark, berries, nuts, resins, flowers, leaves, needles, bulbs, seeds, and peels.

Methods of extraction include:

- Steam distillation (the most common)
- Carbon dioxide gas (CO_2)
- Solvent (absolutes)
- Cold-pressed (scarification)
- Hydro distilled

However, for the home user, the least expensive manner in which to extract the essential oils is either through immersing the ingredients in *another* oil or through alcohol.

The following two recipes/instructions are being provided for their sheer simplicity. There are many methods available to perform these actions. As your skills increase, research additional methods and try new techniques.

Extracting Oils with Oil Method

Oil attracts oil, therefore, one relatively easy way of extracting essential oils is to soak them in oil.

Instructions:

1. In a ceramic crock, add your ingredients.
2. Pour in enough pure olive oil (or safflower oil) to cover the ingredients.
3. Set aside for 24 to 48 hours.
4. Strain the mixture, gently pressing the leaves or flowers to release more oils.
5. Add more fresh flowers or leaves to the already fragrant oil and repeat steps 2-4.
6. Repeat this process an additional six to eight times (or until your essential oil is of the desired strength).
7. Store in tightly sealed bottles in a cool, dark place.

Notes:

Add the oil to whatever you like provided it is for external use. This could be baths, lotions, potpourris, aromatic waters, soaps, or candles.

Extracting Oils with Alcohol Method

Another method of drawing out the plant essence is to soak the ingredients in alcohol. However, when doing so, you should only use alcohol suitable for consumption (undenatured). Do not ever use rubbing alcohol. That being said, the process is the same as the process used when extracting with oils.

Instructions:

1. In a ceramic crock, add your ingredients.
2. Pour in enough alcohol to cover the ingredients.
3. Set aside for 24 to 48 hours.
4. Strain the mixture, gently pressing the leaves or flowers to release more oils.
5. Add more fresh flowers or leaves to the already fragrant alcohol and repeat steps 2-4.
6. Repeat this process an additional six to eight times (or until your essential alcohol/oil meets the desired amount of strength).
7. Store tightly sealed bottles in a cool, dark place.

Notes:

When finished, the fragrant alcohol created can be used as is, or it can be diluted with some water. The extracts created make the base for perfumes because the alcohol evaporates from the skin quickly, thus giving you a blast of fragrance. If you have the need to remove the essence (oil) from the alcohol, simply freeze the container. By doing so, the alcohol will remain a liquid and the essence with be separated and frozen on top of it. Just scrap it off. Using the alcohol method is good for the delicate flowers, as it won't burn the petals as occurs in steam distillation.

Now that we have two basic means for extracting essential oils, the next step is application. There are many methods to choose from in this regard. Depending on the purpose, a person could apply a product containing essential oils by using:

- Massage
- Compresses
- Baths
- Vaporizers
- Sprays

Infused Oils

An infused oil is essentially an oil where the ingredients have been steeped, like a tea, in an oil. This differs from an essential oil in that when making an essential oil you are physically pressing the oil out of the ingredients. An infused oil is simply strained after the ingredients have been suspended in the oil for a few weeks.

Infused oils contain all the healing and health benefits of the herb used. The potency of the oil depends on the herb(s) used and the duration of the infusion. Herbally infused oils can be used for marinades, salad dressings, and in the frying of food. Many people use the infused oils as a base for a variety of products and utilize various methods of application. Some of these products and methods include:

- Bath oils
- Creams
- Salves
- Liniments
- Soap

For making culinary oils choose plant matter and herbs that will enhance your food with a bouquet of flavor. Typical infused oil ingredients for culinary purposes include herbs like rosemary, thyme, basil, chive, garlic, sage, oregano, mild/hot peppers, etc.

For medicinal or beauty oils simply pick your herbs accordingly. For example, lavender smells nice *and* has relaxing and anti-inflammatory properties. You also have a choice as to which natural vegetable oil to use as a carrier oil for your herbal oil infusion. Personal preference reigns supreme in this regard but many infused oil proponents prefer a good high quality cold pressed virgin olive oil for both medicinal and kitchen oils.

There are several ways to make infused oils. However, to get the most taste or healthful benefits from the herb(s) used, the cold infusion method is your best bet.

Cold Infusion Method

1. Gather herbs or flowers.
   a. If using fresh herbs, you need enough to fill the jar. If using dried herbs, the jar is only filled about 1/3 full.
   b. If using fresh herbs, let the herbs sit out in a single layer overnight to wilt. *The herbs must be completely dry before starting your herbal oil. Any moisture will cause spoilage.*
2. Tear or crush the herbs then lightly pack into a clean, sterilized glass jar.
3. Place jar in a small bowl in case of overflow then pour your high quality cold pressed, virgin olive oil (or other natural plant oil) over the herbs.
4. Stir lightly to get rid of any air bubbles.
5. Cap the jar and label it.
6. Store your jar in a cool, dark place (out of direct sunlight) for two to six weeks. If the oil is for kitchen use, just taste your oil until the flavor is where you want it. If you're making a medicinal oil, it's recommended that you infuse for six weeks.

DO **NOT** INFUSE YOUR OIL FOR MORE THAN 6 WEEKS

THE OIL MAY GO RANCID

7. After six weeks or less, strain out the herbs through cheesecloth while expressing oil from the herbs as you go. Repeat the straining process as necessary.
8. Pour the clean, strained oil into a sterile bottle or jar.
9. For longer shelf life, infused oils that you're going to eat should be stored in the refrigerator.

Heat can also be used as a means for creating infused oils. If you are making beauty or medicinal oils, consider adding a 1/2 teaspoon of Vitamin E (per pint) or 15 drops of grapefruit seed extract to preserve them. The following methods are best suited for oil infusions that are ingested.

Oven Infusion Method

1. Place your herbs in an oven safe dish
2. Cover the plant matter with the quality oil of your choice.
3. Cover the dish and place in the oven at 200-degrees (or the lowest possible setting).
4. Cook for three hours.
5. While warm, strain through cheesecloth
6. Squeeze the oil from the herbs as you strain.
7. Pour the oil into a sterile bottle or jar.
8. Allow to cool to room temperature before capping.

Stove Infusion Method

1. Gently simmer oil and plant matter for 2 hours in a double boiler.
2. Strain through cheesecloth.
3. Squeeze the oil from the herbs as you strain.
4. Pour the oil into a sterile bottle or jar.
5. Allow to cool to room temperature before capping.

For stronger infusions, repeat steps 1-2 with the strained oil and a fresh batch of herbs.

Crock-Pot Infusion Method

NOTE: This method can only be used *only* if your crock-pot has a 'warm' or very low setting. In addition, the crock-pot infusion method works well when infusing several oil jars at once.

1. Fill your sterile pint jars with your herbs and oils.
2. Place the jars in the crock-pot, without lids, and cook on low for eight hours.
3. Depending on the size of your crock-pot, you can conceivably handle 3-6 different oils at the same time.
4. Squeeze the oil from the herbs as you strain.
5. Pour the oil into a sterile bottle or jar.
6. Allow to cool to room temperature before capping.

Regardless of which of the infused oil method(s) is/are chosen, you should squeeze any remaining oil from the herbs as you strain. If one of the heating methods is used, you should allow the infusion to cool to room temperature before capping and storing.

The shelf life of the infused oil varies depending on the method that was used, the type of oil, and the storage method. Follow the oil manufacturer recommendations in this regard. It should be noted that the Cold Infusion Method does not heat the oil so you can expect these infusions to have much longer shelf life as compared to an infused oil that warmed/heated the oil.

Chapter 2: Yeast

Why do I need yeast? Well, if you have any desire to generate your own tinctures, you will need alcohol. You have two options when it comes to the alcohol ingredient in a tincture recipe. Either you can buy 80 proof vodka at the store, or you can make it yourself. If you are choosing the latter, you need yeast. If you are a baker extraordinaire, you'll need large quantities of yeast as well.

At this point, it is important to note that yeast naturally occurs in nature on the skin of fruits and vegetables. Well, technically, unless you grew it yourself, a lot of the yeast has been washed off or covered in wax. Therefore, if you want a good yeast, use ingredients that you grew yourself or ingredients that you can trace its sourcing all the back to the grower.

As far as making your own yeast is concerned, luckily, there is a variety of options. Depending on what you want to use the yeast for, whether it be for the aforementioned alcohol generation or for baking, you could do the standard and ubiquitous sourdough starter, you could make a fruit starter, or you could go with potatoes. You can even skip the batter style yeasts and just maintain a bottle of yeast water.

Additionally, you'll need to be mindful as to your future needs and/or potential uses. Meaning, you might not be distilling your own vodka right now, but it might be a good idea to understand how to start, maintain, and dry your own yeast for the use should the need ever arise.

Play around with the provided recipes and the amounts denoted once your yeast is ready. Typically, you'll need about a 1 C of wet starter (batter like substance) in place of 1 packet of yeast. If you've dried your yeast batter, start out by doubling the amount of yeast called for in the recipe. In most cases, a store bought packet of yeast is 1 oz. so you'll need 2 oz. possibly more. The potency of homemade yeast will be a little different from the store-bought version. Also, use different fruit, vegetable, and herb ingredients. The essence of these ingredients will add new and unique flavors to your baked goods.

Lastly, the use of terms/phrases like 'bubbly' or 'bubbling action' refers to the fact that as the yeast begins fermenting it excretes carbon dioxide and alcohol. These excretions cause bubbles to form and stack up in the liquid.

Yeast Water

This is by far the easiest and least labor intensive of the yeast recipes. The reason being, there are only two ingredients. The rest is just time. In addition, the reason the quantities vary is due to the variability in the potentially chosen jar size.

Materials:

Wide mouth Mason Jar (w/ lid)
Cheesecloth (optional)

Ingredients:

1-3 C Sliced Fruit/Vegetable/Herb, leave the skin on as this is where the yeast is located (apples, grapes, cucumbers, raisins, etc.)
2-4 C Filtered or Spring Water (not alkaline or chlorinated – this will kill the yeast)

Instructions:

1. Fill a Mason jar 1/3 to 1/2 full with your chosen fruit, vegetable, or herb.
2. Fill the Mason jar 3/4 full with water (filtered or spring, not alkaline or chlorinated city water).
3. Loosely close the jar, or cover with the cheesecloth, and leave in a warm area (in the sun or by a stove) for approximately 3 days or until a good amount of bubbling has begun forming (this is an indication that the yeast is reacting with the carbohydrates in your fruit, veggie, etc.).
4. Once the bubbling action is well underway, you can begin using the yeast water in your baking recipes.

To use in baking, ignore the specified yeast ingredient and quantity noted in the recipe. Simply insert the yeast water in place of both the yeast and water ingredients but use the recipe specified quantity of water (1 Cup, 2 Cups, etc.).

5. Continue with your recipe as usual.

Fruit Starter

The 'fruit starter' recipe is similar to the yeast water recipe except for this recipe you'll strain out the fruit and add flour. This recipe can be made with most fruits like grapes, apples, plums, peaches, oranges, grapefruits, etc. The key to both of these fruit-laden recipes is to grow and/or harvest (wild) ingredients and to not wash off the fruit. The skins contain the naturally occurring yeast.

Materials:

Medium/Large Glass Bowl
Cheesecloth

Ingredients:

2 C Sliced Fresh Fruit (skin-on)
Filtered or Spring Water for initial fermentation (do not use chlorinated water as it will kill the yeast)
Flour (Use either standard All-Purpose or Whole Wheat. Do not use anything labeled as 'fast rising' or 'bread four')

Instructions:

1. Remove all stems and leaf matter from the fruit and place in a medium to large glass bowl. Do NOT wash the fruit.
2. Crush the fruit buy hand in the bowl, add water until the fruit is submerged about an inch, then cover with cheesecloth.
3. Leave undisturbed for three days.
4. After three days, you should start to see the liquid bubble, indicating that the yeast is growing.
5. Once the bubbling is going strong, strain the liquid that now contains the yeast.
6. Stir in 1 C of flour.
7. Leave your starter at room temperature for 24 hours.
8. Save 1 C of mixture in a separate bowl (to keep the starter going for future use) then add 1 C flour and 1 C water to what remains.
9. Repeat step 8 once a day at the same time for two days. You should have a very bubbly starter at this point.
10. As the mixture is used for baking, just add another cup of flour and water to keep feeding the yeast mixture.

Potato Starter

This yeast starter is quite simple as well. Simply save the water after you boil some potatoes and you're on your way. It is recommended that you not use store bought potatoes for this starter. Read the 'Introduction' in Michael Pollan's book titled *The Omnivore's Dilemma: The Secrets Behind What You Eat* for a perfectly summated reason... chemicals.

Materials:

Medium/Large Glass Bowl
Towel or Cheesecloth

Ingredients:

1 1/2 C Potato Water
1 T Sugar
1-2 C Flour

Instructions:

1. Place the saved potato water in a medium to large glass bowl.
2. Add the sugar and enough flour to make the mixture stiff.
3. Cover and leave overnight in a warm place.
4. If it is nice and bubbly the next morning, you're good to go. If not, you need to begin again with new ingredients.

Sourdough Starter

Materials:

Quart-Sized Wide-Mouth Mason Jars
Cheesecloth

Ingredients:

Water (filtered or spring water, not chlorinated)
Unbleached All Purpose Flour

Instructions:

1. Day 1:
    a. Add 1/2 C flour and 1/2 C water into the Mason jar.
    b. Mix them thoroughly together (should be as thick as pancake batter)
    c. Cover the jar containing the starter with cheesecloth.

2. Day 2:

    a. Add another 1/2 C of flour and as much water as it needs to reach the same pancake batter consistency as seen on Day 1. NOTE: The starter should have a few bubbles in it.
    b. Stir and cover again.

3. Day 3-5:

    a. Starter should be bubblier, possibly with a frothy top.
    b. Add another 1/2 C of flour and as much water as needed to maintain the same pancake batter-like consistency as seen on Day 1 and 2.
    c. Stir and cover again.
    d. Feed the starter about every 24 hours over Days 3-5.
    e. It should always look actively bubbly.

4. Day 6:

    a. The starter should be ready to bake with at this point. NOTE: Altitude and climate (inside and outside) do play a role in the progression of the sourdough starter.

Drying Yeast

Back in the days of westward expansion, one of the challenges faced by many was the making, storing, and transporting of yeast. One of the more widely known stories involving yeast comes from the Book of Exodus when Israelites left Egypt in a hurry. Jews to this day commemorate God's deliverance by abstaining from products with leavening during Passover.

However, if you want to be able to bake bread the instant you arrive (should you find yourself in this situation), then you need to know how to dry and store yeast.

Instructions:

1. Take any of the aforementioned starters and spread it very thinly on a cookie sheet or baking stone.
2. Dehydrate the batter as you would anything else.

NOTE: If you live in a hot and dry climate, you may just be able to cover it with a cheesecloth and place in the sun. You can use a food dehydrator (if you have one) or your oven. The following steps utilize an oven.

3. If you are not in a hot and dry climate, set your oven to the lowest temperature possible and place the cookie sheet or baking stone in the oven.
4. Once the yeast is dry (not browned, burnt, and cooked), you can crumble it and store in an airtight container. NOTE: If the temperature is too high and you cook the yeast, you will have killed the active yeast and rendered the entire batch useless.
5. As with anything homemade, it will last longer if placed in the refrigerator or freezer.

Chapter 3: Vodka

As was discussed in the previous chapter, alcohol, namely 80 proof vodka, is required for making a tincture. Therefore, in an effort to bring the 'ingredients' topic full circle, in lay terms, you need *yeast* to make vodka, and you need *vodka* to make a tincture. This is why the yeast ingredient was discussed first.

Below are some interesting things to note about alcohol:

- Alcohol for human consumption is the same as ethyl alcohol (ethanol) and is usually distilled from grain, potatoes, or fruit. Pure alcohol is about 190 proof, but alcohol bought in stores is usually diluted with distilled water. For comparison, Vodka is pure alcohol diluted to 80 proof.
- All alcohol comes from the fermentation and distillation of a type of grain, including wheat, corn, rice, or rye. Spirits that are called grain alcohols are made from corn, yeast, sugar, and water. Grain alcohol, also known as ethanol, is a twice distilled, neutral spirit with 95% alcohol by volume (ABV) content (or 190-proof).
- Moonshine is an example of an alcohol that is not mellowed. This what gives it its distinctive 'kick'.
- Moonshine made from grain, like corn or rye, is whisky, but alcohol can be made from many different ingredients.
- Corn 'vodka' that comes out of the still at 96% ABV or higher, but doesn't touch oak is still Vodka. Technically, though, it could also be called 'Moonshine'.
- Whiskey can be called 'bourbon' if it is made in the United States and is derived from 51% corn.
- Everclear is 190-proof, meaning, it is 95% alcohol. By comparison, most rum and vodka run between 40% to 60% ABV, or 80 to 120-proof.

Now let's discuss vodka.

The bulk of today's commercially available 80 Proof vodka, depending on which country you live in, is derived from either potatoes or wheat. There are 100 Proof varieties available, but a good tincture will work just fine with an 80 Proof variety.

Poland has long laid claim to the title of being the first purveyors of vodka. However, its original intent was to be used as an aftershave and as an anti-inflammatory medicine for joint pain. It wasn't until the 18th and 19th centuries that its production became commercialized for consumption.

Of course, Russia disputes this.

Regardless, most vodka's are derived from potatoes, grain, or both. If you are more inclined to purchase your vodka instead of making your own, you need to avoid the flavored vodkas and only use neutral vodka. This type of vodka should be labeled as 'classic' or 'regular'.

The key to creating a potato-derived vodka is to use the malted grains as the necessary enzyme to break down the starch of the potato into basic sugars. The information noted in the following recipe *was* located on the "Home Distillation of Alcohol" website. Unfortunately, that site is no longer in existence.

Before the website came down though, the administrator/operator posted some emails from a fellow distiller where the two discussed the recipe. I have edited that conversation for the sake of readability.

Part I: 80 Proof Potato Vodka (Stepped Infusion Mash)

A 'stepped infusion mash' is where you start the saccharification process at a low temperature and then move it up in steps, halting for a certain time period at each step to give each enzyme time to break down as much as they can at each stage. If you have made beer in the past using an all-grain mash you will understand the process.

Ingredients:

1/2 kg (1.10 lbs) Sprouted Malted Ale Barley (or Sprouted Standard
    Malted Barley)
3-4 kg (6.61-8.81 lbs) Potatoes
Water (enough to cover potatoes + 2-3" for evaporation)
Yeast

Instructions:

1. Cook your potatoes so they are still stiff - about 12- 15 minutes at med-high heat. Up to 20 minutes at low heat. (Note they should still be a bit undercooked, definitely not soft, mushy, or floury.)
2. Add coarsely milled barley where the particles are about 1/16 to 3/32" in size. (Do not use fine milled.)
3. Cover with sufficient water and bring to 113 F (45 C). Hold 15 minutes stirring regularly.
4. Bring up to 133 F (56 C). Hold 15 minutes stirring regularly
5. Bring up to 149 F (65 C). Hold 15 minutes stirring constantly.
6. Bring up to 158 F (70 C). Hold 15 minutes stirring constantly.

Added all up, Steps 3 through 6 (once Step 3 reaches a boil), takes one hour. This should suffice for a small batch. Some batches will take longer especially bigger batches. Most of the liquefaction and saccharification occurs in Steps 5 and 6 rather than Steps 3 and 4. If you want to alter this, reduce Steps 3 and 4 to 10 minutes and increase Steps 5 and 6 to 20 minutes or longer where required.

7. Once virtually all the starch is liquefied, and broken down to simple sugars, you need to halt the enzymatic process by raising the temperature to 176 F (80 C) (aka Mashing Out) and then drop it back as quickly as possible to between 140 F (60 C) and 122 F (50 C) so the sugars don't get scorched or burnt. [*A refrigerator or chest freezer with a wireless digital thermometer can accomplish this.*]
8. Cool down further to 75 F (24 C), establish a specific gravity (SG) of 1060 (min) to 1080 (max = ideal), add the yeast and begin fermentation.

Make minute adjustments to the basic formula with each batch by adjusting the temperature and time (duration) allows you to get a feel for the process and expand your knowledge base rapidly via hands on experimentation as opposed to reading a book.

It is highly recommended that you start with small batches, as was noted in the ingredients list. What you want is plenty of enzymes together from a small batch but 'brewed' in a large pot to prevent boiling over. Once you have this basic process under control, and gained a bit of experience, you can reduce the number of steps further thus saving time and energy while producing virtually the same result.

So, that's what the email exchange essentially had to say. Now, are you ready for the bad news?

Sadly, the generation of the mash is only 'Part I' of a three part process. The next two Parts are the 'Fermentation' and 'Distilling' processes. I only provide Part I here as an example so if you're tempted to make your own, you'll have some idea of what to expect in terms of the time commitment and material list. No one ever said making vodka was a short process. As with all things worthwhile, it takes time and patience.

For a complete breakdown of all three Parts, complete with steps, ingredients, and parts lists, I recommend you visit the Mile Hi Distilling website and read everything they have to say on the "How to Make Vodka: A Distillers Guide" page. It will help you immensely. [Full URL: https://milehidistilling.com/how-to-make-vodka/]

Be sure to read the entire page because the information pertaining to foreshots, heads, hearts, and tails is vitally important.

Publisher's Note

Distilling can be a dangerous enterprise and should not be undertaken lightly. Alcohol distilling is volatile by nature and the end-product can have side effects that could potentially be harmful as well. Moreover, there may also be local, state, and federal laws that prohibit the creation of spirits in your locality. Check to see if any of these laws are applicable in your area. The 'mash' recipe and accompanying URLs has been provided solely for example and informational purposes only. The author and publisher assume no liability for a reader's attempted use or misuse of the information being provided. Please consult with experienced professionals and/or seek instruction from certified and credentialed instructors knowledgeable in such matters before undertaking this or any potentially dangerous endeavor.

Chapter 4: Ingredients

As you begin working your way through the recipes contained in each of the subsequent chapters, you'll notice that most of these recipes require, more or less, ingredients that are somewhat readily available in nature. The following is not an exhaustive list by any means, but it will give you a good foundation of understanding when making your assorted remedies.

Potential Ingredients

Activated Charcoal

Used for acute cases of food poisoning, intestinal illness, vomiting, diarrhea, and the ingestion of toxins, etc. Caution should be used, as activated charcoal can be a toxin as well. Consult with your medical professional as this ingredient may interact with Tylenol and your heart and depression medications.

Anise Hyssop

Anise hyssop makes a delightful addition to mixed herbal teas and a fine tea all to itself. It has a delicate anise or licorice flavor. The tea is naturally sweet, so extra sweetener is not necessary. In fact, the tea is so sweet that it can be used to sweeten other foods. Folklore medicine employed anise hyssop herbal tea to treat colds, coughs, and fevers, to induce sweating, and to strengthen a weak heart.

Amaranth

This ingredient is high in (plant) proteins that the body quickly and easily breaks down into amino acids then reforms the amino acids into usable proteins. The reformed proteins are essential for growth, the creation of new cells and tissues, immediate energy, and metabolic functionality. The anti-inflammatory properties of amaranth can also help to alleviate conditions like arthritis, gout, and other inflammation-related issues. Also contains a high concentration of calcium. There are very few leafy vegetables that contain higher levels of calcium, making amaranth a veritable superfood in terms of boosting bone strength and preventing osteoporosis.

Arnica

Topical cream used for muscle pain or injury, bruises or any type of trauma. Reduces healing time for bruises and sore muscles if applied right after the injury occurs. Note: This is not to be ingested or rubbed in open wounds.

Borage

Several parts of this plant are useful in the kitchen! Young leaves can be added to salads, and the blue flowers can be candied, used as a garnish, or added to drinks. Borage is very good in teas. In modern herbalism, Borage is said to be effective against weak or diminished adrenal function, fevers, inflammation, sore and inflamed eyes, colds, bronchitis, chronic catarrh, congestion, pleurisy, and fever.

Calendula

Calendula species have been used traditionally as culinary and medicinal herbs for centuries. Fresh petals can be used in salads, dried petals can be used to color cheese and as a replacement for saffron. A yellow dye can also be extracted from the flowers. Calendula ointments can be used for minor cuts, burns, and skin irritation. The oil is used medicinally as an anti-inflammatory and a remedy for healing wounds. Lab studies suggest that Calendula extracts have antiviral, antigenotoxic (prevents genetic damage within a cell), and anti-inflammatory properties. In herbalism, Calendula ingredients in a suspension or tincture is used topically for treating acne, reducing inflammation, controlling bleeding, soothing irritated tissue, abdominal cramps, and constipation. It should be noted though that Calendula are known to cause allergic reactions and therefore this herb should be avoided during pregnancy.

Catnip

This self-sowing annual is a good host for attracting beneficial insects and keeps mosquitoes at bay in gardens therefore making it a good insect repellent. Catnip is a vigorous growing mint loved by cats. This is beneficial for homesteaders and farmers where cats are engaged to keep mice at bay. It is brewed into a tea to treat colds, headaches, flu, and fever. Tea also has a relaxing effect on children.

Cayenne Powder

Though this is a good addition to many foods, it is even better to have in a medicine cabinet. Topically, cayenne powder helps stop bleeding rapidly. I've read cases of it being taken internally during heart attacks to increase blood flow and help clear blockage, though thankfully, I've never had to test this one. It is also a useful remedy to take internally during illness as it increases blood flow and speeds recovery. Cayenne is most widely regarded as a circulatory stimulant said to strengthen the heart and blood vessels while promoting increased vitality.

See Chapter 10 for additional information related to cayenne as an ingredient.

Chamomile

Chamomile flower tea is one of the most consumed teas in the world behind regular black tea. Chamomile flowers have a naturally sweet taste with a hint of an apple flavor. Chamomile is a good herbal source of Magnesium, and is known as a soothing and relaxing herb. It makes an excellent tea in the evening or in times of stress because of its mildly sedative and soothing properties. It is an excellent herb for children especially when teething and can even be an effective remedy for pink eye. Rubbing the cooled tea on the stomach of colicky infants helps sooth them as well. Chamomile can be made into a tincture for a more potent effect. A tincture will also extend the shelf life. Avoid chamomile if you are allergic to ragweed.

Comfrey

Promotes healing from injuries and broken bones. Combining comfrey with plantain in a salve/poultice can greatly reduce the healing time and help prevent and reverse infection. Works well on bug bites, cuts, bruises, and poison ivy.

Culver's Root

Also known as Bowman's Root, this root has also been used as a tonic to treat liver and gallbladder disorders and to promote healthy bile flow. Culver's root is a native North American plant that is well established in Native American herbal medicine. In the Southern U.S., it is still used extensively as a tonic for the stomach and a blood purifier and is known as Black Root. Culver's extract has also been used effectively for diarrhea, chronic constipation, indigestion, sallow complexion, and dull frontal headaches.

Echinacea

Native Americans have used echinacea for hundreds of years as a means to treat infections, wounds, and as a general "cure all." Historically, echinacea has been used to treat everything from scarlet fever, syphilis, and malaria to blood poisoning, and diphtheria. Echinacea contains active substances that enhance the activity of the immune system, relieve pain, reduce inflammation, and have hormonal, antiviral, and antioxidant effects.

Eucalyptus Herb and Essential Oil

Addresses respiratory issues related to congestion or sinus troubles. Can easily be added to a salve and rubbed on the chest like a vapor-rub for coughing and respiratory illness.

Feverfew

Tanacetum parthenium, known as feverfew or bachelor's buttons, is a flowering plant in the daisy family Asteraceae. A traditional medicinal herb is commonly used for prevention and treatment of migraine headaches, fevers, rheumatoid arthritis, stomachaches, toothaches, insect bites, infertility, and problems with menstruation and labor during childbirth.

Garlic

Considered a natural wonder drug, garlic is useful for drawing toxins and impurities out of the body. It is also used to for treating and prevent gum disease, addressing common cold and flu symptoms, yeasts infections and soothing yeast infection discomfort, heal cold sores, and the oil helps remove splinters.

Ginger

Ginger is great for nausea, reflux, stomach trouble, and morning sickness. It also works well for motion sickness and is soothing to the stomach after a digestive illness or food poisoning. This medicinal root is highly regarded for its antioxidant, antibacterial, and antiviral properties. It also contains anti-inflammatory properties, which makes it a valuable natural remedy ingredient when combating headaches, migraines, joint pain, and menstrual problems.

Hyssop

The bright blue flowers of this member of the mint family add lovely color to your herb garden! Leaves may be brewed into a tea with soothing and medicinal properties for colds, flu, sore throat, bruises, and burns. It is also said to be effective as an expectorant and to promote improved circulation and digestion.

Lemon Balm

Strongly lemon scented, Lemon Balm is a popular ingredient of herbal teas and potpourris! Fresh leaves give a nice lemon flavor to salads, soups, sauces, and meats. Lemon Balm is also valued for its medicinal properties! Used to treat colds, flu, indigestion, etc.

Mad-Dog Skullcap

Herbalists claim it is an effective headache remedy, great for insomnia and both calms and strengthens the nervous system. Flowering tops of skullcap are used in daily teas as well as formulas for chronic conditions. Called Mad-dog because the tea was once used as a folk remedy for rabies. Enjoy its numerous small blue flowers from July through September or put the leaves in a pillow to induce restful sleep.

Mint

Second only to Chamomile in popularity among herbal teas. Peppermint tea soothes the digestive track and is helpful for heartburn, nausea, morning sickness, and indigestion. Peppermint is a delicious tea, but it can be consumed either by itself or with other herbs to help increase each ingredient's effectiveness.

Moringa Tree

Nicknamed the 'Tree of Life' and the 'Miracle Tree', nearly every aspect of the Moringa tree can be harvested, eaten, and steeped to access the wide assortment of medicinal properties. The Moringa tree contains vitamin A, B, C, E, and K, protein, amino acids, beta-carotene, and manganese. It aids in the reduction of blood sugar levels, is rumored to slow aging, regulate hormonal imbalances, reduce swelling, boost the immune system, and increase breast milk production. These trees are highly regarded for rapid growth, generally sprouting within a week, and dwarf varieties can be grown indoors in pots with ease. Additionally, both the gum and bark can be eaten as a means to accessing its assorted healing properties.

Myrrh

This tree gum is usually ground into a powder and added as an ingredient in antiseptics for mouthwashes, gargles, tooth powders, toothaches, and toothpastes. To be used as a tincture mouthwash, it is usually combined with borax. Myrrh is also used in some liniments and healing salves that may be applied to abrasions, minor skin ailments, bruises, aches, and sprains. Veterinarians use myrrh for healing wounds as well. Myrrh gum is commonly claimed to remedy indigestion, ulcers, colds, cough, asthma, lung congestion, arthritis pain, and cancer. This ingredient is also recommended for rheumatic, arthritic, and circulatory problems, and for menstrual cramps, menopause, and uterine tumors.

Oat Berry

Oat berries (sometimes referred to as 'groats') are the hulled kernels of the cereal grain oat. Berries can also be harvested from other cereal grains like wheat, rye, and barley. Groats are whole grains that include the cereal germ and the fiber-rich bran portion of the grain. Oat berries, in particular, have a range of potential health benefits. Oats are loaded with dietary fiber and the possible health benefits include reducing the risk of coronary artery disease, lowering levels of cholesterol, and reducing one's risk of colorectal cancer.

Passionflower

Passionflower is a climbing vine that is native to the southeastern United States, and Central and South America. Take passionflower by mouth for insomnia, anxiety, attention deficit-hyperactivity disorder (ADHD), pain symptoms, fibromyalgia, opioid withdrawal symptoms, reducing anxiety and nervousness (calming), muscle spasms, and heart failure. Passionflower can be applied directly to the skin for hemorrhoids, burns, and swelling (inflammation).

Peppermint Herb and Essential Oil

Another great digestive herb. For upset stomach or digestive illness, the herb is made into a tea. The tincture can be used internally or externally for headache or digestive troubles and when combined with a few other digestive herbs, it makes a highly effective digestive aid and nausea remedy. The essential oil applied behind the ears and on the feet helps alleviate headache or nausea and a weak tea made from the herb and rubbed on the skin can help sooth a colicky baby. This herb can be used in the essential oil for homemade toothpaste.

Plantain

A natural remedy for poultices addressing infections, poison ivy, cuts, scrapes, bites, and bee stings. Combine plantain and comfrey in a poultice to keep bites from eating away any tissue and help to site heal completely.

Raspberry Leaf

Highly nutritious and is good for the balancing of hormones and as a skin rejuvenator. This leaf is often consumed during pregnancy as it can strengthen the uterus and contains Magnesium, Potassium, and B-Vitamins. Tea's incorporating this ingredient taste similar to black tea. Herbalists recommend this tincture and/or tea to treat infertility, painful periods (menses), endometriosis, and Polycystic Ovary Syndrome (PCOS).

Rosemary

This fragrant herb originates from the Mediterranean, and most people associate it with cooking. However, rosemary has many health benefits as well. The herb is rich in calcium, iron, and vitamin B6, and has a potent effect on the nervous and digestive systems. Rosemary is also high in carnosic acid, which serves to aid sleep by cleansing the mind of toxins. This herb can also be applied topically for soothing skin inflammation if added to a carrier oil like olive oil or coconut oil before applying. Rosemary oil extract may cause irritation and inflammation of the skin if applied to open wounds.

Slippery Elm

Helpful for sore or irritated throats and for loss of voice. Include this herb in tinctures or teas for sore throat relief.

St. John's Wort

St. John's Wort is most commonly used for depression and symptoms that sometimes go along with mood such as nervousness, tiredness, poor appetite, and trouble sleeping. Caution should be used with this ingredient as St. John's Wort might cause serious interactions with some medications.

Tarragon

This healing herb can help treat stomachaches, toothaches, and insomnia. Tarragon could also help improve insulin sensitivity and help regulate blood sugar. It can also help normalize sleep patterns and reduce pain associated with Osteoarthritis, as well as sparking an increase in appetite.

Thyme

Thyme is a Mediterranean herb used to treat diarrhea, stomachaches, arthritis, and sore throats. This herb is also thought to have natural antibacterial, insecticidal, and antifungal properties in addition to aiding in the reduction of high blood pressure. Thyme might protect people from colon cancers and wild thyme has caused cell death in breast cancer cells. The essential oil of thyme also addresses the fungus present in oral and vaginal yeast infections.

Turmeric

This bright orange spice is the only source of the powerful antioxidant, curcumin. The curcumin component is harvested from the dried rhizome or root cuttings. Curcumin has been used by herbalists for thousands of years as it has been found to reduce joint and muscle inflammation and arthritis stiffness. It may also be beneficial for enhancing brain health and function and in fighting certain cancers, depression, and Alzheimer's.

Witch Hazel (Winterbloom)

The leaves and bark of the North American witch hazel may be used to produce a cooling agent. Once decocted, witch hazel was widely used by Native Americans, but today its tannins are mainly used externally on hemorrhoids to shrink blood vessels, minor bleeding, and skin irritations. It makes a great skin toner and is good for postpartum bottom. Today, witch hazel is typically sold in pharmacies as 'witch hazel water' and is included as an ingredient in semisolid ointments, creams, gels, and salves.

Yarrow

Yarrow has been used to induce sweating and to stop bleeding wounds. It also has been reported to reduce heavy menstrual bleeding and pain. It has been used to relieve GI ailments, for cerebral and coronary thromboses, to lower high blood pressure, to improve circulation, and to tone varicose veins.

Additional Ingredients

These ingredients aren't necessarily herbal in nature, but can either be made by you or procured (bought) as manufactured products in a store. Their inclusion in your 'medicine cabinet' can be beneficial at times.

Aloe Vera Plant and Liquid

Can be grown in your own home to treat burns (water scalding or fire), sunburns, and blisters.

Apple Cider Vinegar

Can be used for digestive troubles, indigestion, food poisoning and more. Taken in a dose of 1 teaspoon per 8 ounces of water every hour, it helps shorten the duration of any type of illness.

Baking Soda

Can be used for severe heartburn or urinary tract infections. Ingesting a 1/4 teaspoon straight or in a little water can alleviate symptoms quickly. It can also be made into a poultice and used on spider bites.

Coconut Oil

Can be used as a skin salve, diaper cream, makeup remover, and antifungal treatment. Can be used to apply tinctures and help aid absorption externally and for dry skin and chapped lips. There is also growing evidence that daily consumption of 1/4 cup or more of coconut oil can help protect against Alzheimer's and nourish the thyroid.

Epsom Salt

Good as a bath soak for sore muscles. Dissolved in water, it can also be a good soak to help remove splinters.

Gelatin

During any type of illness, after surgery, or when there is a cut that might scar, gelatin can be used to speed the healing of the skin. There is evidence that it is also effective in improving blood clotting when used externally on a wound.

Homemade Neosporin

Used on cuts, bruises, rashes and anything else antibiotic ointment could be used on. See the Homemade Neosporin recipe in Chapter 8.

Hydrogen Peroxide

Can be used in homemade OxyClean and for cleaning out wounds. Be careful about overuse though. The first time it is used it will clean the wound. Repeated use will prevent the wound from closing. Dilute peroxide 1-1 with water to handle excessive wax build up. Be warned though, excessive time in the ear canal (on tissue) can cause irritation and fungal infections.

Probiotics

Used during, and after, any illness to repair and restore gut bacteria. Additional uses, and potential value added side effects, include improved skin conditions (with regular use), pregnancy, and children who seem to have a constant illness or ear infections. Probiotics are recommended for pregnant mothers as babies in utero receive their gut bacteria from their mother. If taken during pregnancy, it can make a tremendous difference in whether or not the baby will get ear infections or illness in the first months. If the mother opts to not ingest during pregnancy then they can be administered post birth should sickness arise.

Vitamin C

Helpful for all illnesses, but especially flu-related illnesses. In powder form, it is additive free and can be mixed into food or drinks.

Chapter 5: General Home Remedies

These general home remedy recipes represent 'olde tyme' methods for addressing specific ailments. I have separated the 'ailment' recipes out from all of the other topics (tinctures, salves, poultices, etc.). This was done because, as you will see, the ingredients lists don't really fit into any of the other categories as neatly as they should given the purist definition of a tincture, salve, or poultice.

Meaning, the recipes are not capturing the essential oils from various plants or herbs (tincture), or rubbing something on the skin (salve), or rubbing something on and covering with bandaging (poultice).

Be advised, some of the recipes do contain tincture liquids. The recipe assumes you already have the tincture on hand and are not making the tincture. That being said, if you need the tincture to complete the home remedy recipe, every effort was made to locate said tincture recipe and it has been included in Chapter 9: Tinctures.

Animal Gatorade

Treatments:
Pet and livestock dehydration.

Ingredients:
2 qt. Water
4 oz. Honey, or Karo syrup
1 t Salt
1 t Soda

Instructions:
1. Combine ingredients and mix well.
2. Administer to small animals with eyedropper. (Dogs and cats may drink it on their own.)

Anti-Fungal / Anti-Yeast Treatment

Treatments:
Fungus and yeast issues as well as athlete's foot.

Ingredients:
2 T Boric Acid
1 C Cornstarch

Instructions:
1. Combine ingredients in a large salt shaker.
2. Shake on any area with fungal rash.

Dosage:
Apply one to two times daily as needed until healed. Please note that some skin rashes that are severe enough may take up to two weeks to heal.

Arthritis Drink

Treatments:
Arthritis related pain.

Ingredients:
1/3 C Honey
1 C Vinegar
16 oz. Grape Juice
32 oz. Apple Juice

Instructions:
1. Combine all ingredients.

Dosage:
Drink 1 or 2 ounces daily.

Notes:
Once the drink is sufficiently combined, it can be frozen for future use.

Cough Drops

Treatments:
Cough due to cold.

Ingredients:
1 C Sugar
1/2 C Water
1 T Lemon Juice (fresh)
1 T Honey
1/2 t Ginger (ground)
1/4 t Cloves(ground)

Instructions:
1. Combine all ingredients in a pan over medium heat.
2. Allow to simmer while stirring.
3. Once simmering, reduce heat to low and stir.
4. Allow to simmer on low for 15-20 minutes stirring regularly.
5. Remove from heat and allow the mixture to cool for 5 minutes. (Mixture should be thick, dark, and syrupy.)
6. Line a baking tray with parchment paper then spoon the mixture onto the parchment in lozenge size dollops (small quarters).
7. Cover with a light dusting of powdered sugar.
8. Shuffle the lozenge's around to get a good coating of the powdered sugar.
9. Store in a parchment lined tin or Tupperware container away from heat.

Dosage:
Take one lozenge as needed.

Notes:
Lozenges can be added to hot water to make a tea as well.

Cold and Flu

Recipe #1 - Season Helper (for colds)

Ingredients:
1/4 t Ginger (powder)
1/4 t Cayenne Pepper
1 T Honey
1 T Apple Cider Vinegar
2 T Hot Water

Instructions:
Combine all ingredients to make a tea.

Dosage:
1. Take one teaspoon every hour.

Notes:
The cayenne pepper really gets things moving in the sinus, as this stuff is potent, but not unbearable.

Recipe #2 – Tea for Season (cough and cold)

Ingredients:
5 slices of Ginger
1 Garlic Clove (sliced)
1-2 T Lemon Juice (fresh)
Honey (to taste)

Instructions:
1. Combine all ingredients in a large mug then cover with boiling water.
2. Let it steep for 5 minutes then sip until gone.

Dosage:
Several cups throughout the day (3-4) until symptoms abate.

Dakin's Solution

Treatments:
Kills most bacteria's and viruses.

Ingredients:
4 C Water
1/2 t Baking Soda
5.25% Sodium Hypochlorite Solution (unscented bleach)

Instructions:
1. Wash your hands well with soap and water.
2. Measure out 32 ounces (4 cups) of clean water. Pour into a clean pan and allow water to boil for 15 minutes.
3. Remove pan from heat.
4. Using a sterile measuring spoon, add 1/2 tsp. of baking soda to the water.
5. Measure bleach according to the strength that is desired:
   - Full strength – add 3 oz. bleach
   - 1/2 strength – add 3 T + 1/2 t
   - 1/4 strength – add 1 T +2 t
   - 1/8 strength – add 2 1/2 t
6. Place the solution in a jar and close it tightly with a sterile lid. Cover the closed jar with tin foil to protect it from sunlight.
7. This solution can be made and kept for up to a month. Discard any unused portion of the antiseptic each month and make a new batch.

Notes:
Can be used on minor scrapes, skin and tissue infections, before and after surgical procedures, as a mouthwash (do not swallow), wound irrigation solution, and it can be applied as a wet-to-moist dressing. The body's wound-healing tissues and fluids can decrease the antibacterial effect. Therefore, use this daily for minor wounds and twice daily for heavily draining or contaminated wounds. Protect the surrounding healthy skin with a moisture barrier ointment (i.e. petroleum jelly) or skin sealant as needed to prevent irritation.

Dandelion Wine

Treatments:
Liver function and maintenance.

Ingredients:
3-5 Q Dandelion Blossoms
5 Q Water
3 lbs Sugar
1 Orange + rind from avg sized orange (organic only, omit if not)
1 Lemon + rind from avg sized lemon (organic only, omit if not)
1 pkg (8 g) live yeast
Whole Wheat Bread

Instructions:
1. Find a field of dandelions in bloom. (Hint: follow the bees).
2. Pick dandelions with a sweeping motion of your parted fingers, like a comb (leave green sepals, discard stalks).
3. Put the blossoms immediately into a large crock-pot/glass mixing bowl/plastic container.
4. Boil the water and then pour it over flowers.
5. Cover your crock/bowl/container with cheesecloth.
6. Stir daily for three days.
7. On the fourth day, strain blossoms from liquid.
8. Cook strained liquid with sugar and rinds for 30-60 minutes.
9. Return the cooked liquid to the crock/bowl/container and add citrus juice.
10. When liquid has cooled to blood temperature, soften yeast, spread on toast, and float toast in crock/bowl/container.
11. Cover and let the yeast work for two days.
12. After two days, strain the liquid again.
13. Return strained liquid to the crock/bowl/container for one day and allow it to settle again.
14. Filter into very clean bottles and cork lightly.
15. Don't drink until winter solstice.

Notes:
A week of work yields a drink that's good for your liver, as well.

Dandruff

Ingredients:
2 T Shampoo (non dandruff)
3 drops Tea Tree Oil

Instructions:
1. Add the tea tree oil to your regular shampoo, mix well, and apply to wet hair in the shower as usual.

Deodorant (Wet)

Ingredients:
1 t Baking Soda
Few drops of Water (to thickness you desire)
Couple drops of Coconut Oil
Couple drops of any Fragrant Essential Oil

Instructions:
1. Mix all ingredients together.

Deodorant Powder (Dry)

Ingredients:
1 part Orris Root
1 part Orange Peel Powder
1 part Lemon Peel Powder

Instructions:
1. Mix equal parts of all ingredients.
2. Put mixture into a powder dispenser and use on any part of the body to deodorize.

Notes:
To add a little sent to the powder, considering including calamus root or licorice root.

Ear Infection

Recipe #1 – Garlic

<u>Ingredients:</u>
1 Clove of Garlic

<u>Instructions:</u>
1. Peel the skin from a bud of garlic then cut to fit the outside of the ear canal.
2. Wrap in a piece of gauze, heat gently.
3. Insert into the canal.

Recipe #2 – Mullein Oil

<u>Ingredients:</u>
3-5 drops of Mullein Oil

<u>Instructions:</u>
1. Place a few drops of mullein oil on a cotton ball.
2. Gently place in the ear canal.

Recipe #3 – Assorted Oils

<u>Treatments:</u>
Infections and earaches.

<u>Ingredients:</u>
1 t Mullein Oil
1 t Garlic Oil
1 t Calendula Oil
1 t St. John's Wort Oil

<u>Instructions:</u>
1. Mix ingredients in a brown bottle that has a built in dropper lid.
2. Shake well to mix.
3. Before bed, fill your ear canal with a dropper or two full.
4. Insert a cotton ball to keep the liquid from running out.
5. Repeat nightly as needed.

Recipe #4 – Yarrow Leaves

Treatments:
Ear infection.

Ingredients:
Yarrow Leaves

Instructions:
1. Steep yarrow leaves in warm water.
2. Pour the warm liquid into the ear canal to soothe and reduce infection.

Recipe #5 – Herb Infusion

Treatments:
Ear infection.

Ingredients:
Anti-Inflammatory/Bacterial Herbs

Instructions:
1. Anti-inflammatory and antibacterial herbs (chamomile, echinacea, golden rod, and golden seal) can be taken internally or infused and dropped into the ear canal.

First-Aid Eyewash

Treatments:
Eye irritants, exposure to chemicals.

Ingredients:
1 T Comfrey Root
1 T Fennel Seed
4 oz. Water

Instructions:
1. Place the ingredients in pot and heat for a few minutes.
2. Remove from heat and allow to steep until cool.
3. Strain carefully through a fine textured fabric and refrigerate.

Notes:
Always keep this formula in the refrigerator and remake it every 3 days as needed.

Gallstones (Cholesterol)

Treatments:
Gallstones due to cholesterol.

Ingredients:
8 quarts Apple Juice
4 quarts Apple Cider
Mild Homemade Laxatives (Epsom salts and olive oil)

Instructions:
Mix 1 1/3 C apple juice and 2/3 C apple cider.

Dosage:
Drink the combined 2 C mix daily for six days.

Hand Sanitizer

Treatments:
Hand sanitation.

Ingredients:
1 C Aloe Vera Gel
1 t Rubbing Alcohol
2 t Vegetable Glycerin
8-10 drops Tea Tree Essential Oil (or Lavender Essential Oil)

Instructions:
1. Simply blend all of the ingredients together and store.

Hand Warmer

Treatments:
General coldness of extremities.

Ingredients:
25 g Iron Powder (filings or grindings)
1 g Salt (Sodium Chloride)
1 T Vermiculite
1 t Water

Instructions:
1. Combine iron powder and salt in a plastic bag, shake to mix.
2. Add vermiculite (or charcoal or sawdust), shake to mix.
3. Store in airtight jar until ready to use.

TO ACTIVATE,
1. Add water, seal the bag tight, then squeeze and shake.

Notes:
Fine steel wool could be used instead of iron filings.

Hardtack

Ingredients:
3 C Flour
2 t Salt
1 C Water

Instructions:
1. In a large bowl, mix flour and salt then add water and stir (or work with hands) to blend.
2. Knead the dough, adding more flour if mixture becomes too sticky.
3. Turn out onto a floured board and roll the dough into a rectangle about 1/2 inch thick
4. Using a sharp knife, cut dough into 3 inch squares.
5. Using clean nail, poke 16 holes though each square.
6. Bake at 375-degrees for 25 minutes or until brown.
7. Store in an airtight container.

Hemorrhoid Treatment

Treatments:
Hemorrhoids and postpartum bottom.

Ingredients:
Undistilled Witch Hazel
Cotton Balls

Instructions:
1. Drench a cotton ball with undistilled witch hazel.
2. Press against the hemorrhoid or swollen blood vessel.
3. Repeat 2-3 times a day until condition lessens.

Ice Pack

Treatments:
Bruising, swelling, twisted ankles.

Ingredients:
2 C Water
1/3 C Alcohol (80 proof - rubbing alcohol, vodka, etc.)
Plastic Bag (zipper top)

Instructions:
1. Combine water and alcohol in a zipper top plastic bag.
2. Seal the top and freeze.

Notes:
The alcohol keeps it from freezing solid and creates a gel - like ice pack.

Insomnia / Relaxation Formula

Ingredients:
2 T Valerian
2 T Yarrow
2 T Lavender
3 T Spearmint
3 T Catnip

Instructions:
1. Mix all ingredients together.
2. Put in a jar and label accordingly.

Dosage:
Combine 1 T per cup of hot water then steep for 15 minutes. Strain liquid through cloth and drink.

Jock Itch

Treatments:
Itching, burning sensation of the groin.

Ingredients:
2 oz. Coconut Oil
2 oz. Neem Oil
1 oz. Apple Cider Vinegar
10 drops Lavender Essential Oil
5 drops Tea Tree Oil
3 drops Oregano Oil (optional)

Instructions:
1. Combine all of the **oil** ingredients only in a glass jar.
2. Once combined, blend in the Apple Cider Vinegar to create a cream.

Dosage:
Rub onto the affected area twice daily.

Notes:
For a cooling sensation, keep the ointment refrigerated.

Kidney Stone Tea

Treatments:
Kidney stones.

Ingredients:
2 t Hydrangea Root
1 t Wild Yam Root
1 t Cramp Bark
1 1/2 quarts Water
1 t Joe Pye Weed
1/2 t Corn Silk
1/2 t Plantain Leaf
1/2 t Yarrow Leaf
30 drops Shepherd's Purse Tincture (if bleeding occurs)

Instructions:
1. Add hydrangea, wild yam and cramp bark to water in a saucepan.
2. Bring to a boil, then turn down heat and simmer for 15 minutes.
3. Remove from heat, add other herbs, cover pan and steep for at least 20 minutes.
4. Strain and keep refrigerated.

Dosage:
Drink 3 to 4 C daily. If bleeding occurs, add 30 drops shepherd's purse tincture to each cup of tea.

Notes:
[1] A tea is especially appropriate when treating a kidney infection because you should already be drinking plenty of water to keep kidneys flushed and help prevent the stones from forming. For convenience, you can also take this formula as a tincture; take 2 to 3 dropperfuls a day.

[2] See Chapter 10 – Additional Information for more information on kidney stone treatment.

Low Libido

Recipe #1 – Love Motion Potion

Ingredients:
1/2 oz. Damiana
1/2 oz. Siberian Ginseng
1/2 oz. Ashwagandha
1/8 oz. Licorice Root
1/2 oz. Prickly Ash Bark
1 1/2 pints Water

Instructions:
1. Mix the herbs well.
2. Bring 1 1/2 pints of water to a boil.
3. Add the herbs and simmer for five minutes over very low heat/flame.
4. Strain the simmered liquid.
5. Serve hot or iced.

Notes:
This tea invigorates your senses, uplifts your spirits, gets your juices flowing, and is geared for both men and women. This tea can be quite energizing, so drink it in the evening ONLY if you are planning some exciting late night activities!

Recipe #2 – Love Tea

Ingredients:
2 C Water
1/2 oz. Rose Petals (liquid)
1/2 oz. Spearmint (liquid)
1/8 oz. Licorice Root (liquid)
1/2 oz. Hawthorn Herb (liquid
Pinch of Coriander
Pinch of Cinnamon
Pinch of Nutmeg
1/4 t Vanilla Extract

Instructions:
1. Boil two cups of water.
2. Once boiling, pour liquid rose petals, spearmint, licorice root, and hawthorn herb in water.
3. Once incorporated, stir in the pinch of coriander, cinnamon, nutmeg, and add a touch of vanilla to taste.
4. Cover and turn heat down to simmer for three minutes.
5. Take the tea off the heat, stir, and let stand for five minutes.
6. Pour into mugs and sit with your loved one for a nice conversation while sipping tea. Let things go from there.

NOTE: Adjust the amount of the liquid ingredients (Rose Petals, Spearmint, Licorice Root, and Hawthorn Herb) as needed to achieve the desired result.

Mosquito And Tick Repellent

Treatments:
Mosquito and tick repellent.

Ingredients:
1 C Spring Water
1/2 C Lemon Juice
15 drops Peppermint Oil
10 drops Lavender Oil

Instructions:
1. Add all ingredients in a clean spray bottle and shake.
2. Store in the refrigerator.

Notes:
Shake well before each use. Can be used on dogs.

Mouthwash

Recipe #1 – Patricia Davis' Mouthwash

Ingredients:
250 ml Cheap Brandy
30 drops Peppermint Essential Oil
20 drops Thyme Essential Oil
10 drops Myrrh Essential Oil
10 drops Fennel Essential Oil

Instructions:
1. Combine all ingredients, mix well.
2. Store in airtight bottle.

Recipe #2 – Mint

Ingredients:
1 C Water
1/4 C Plain Soda Drink
4 t Vegetable Glycerin
1 t Aloe Vera Gel
10 drops Peppermint Essential Oil (or spearmint or Pudinhara)

Instructions:
1. Boil the water and then add the soda, glycerin, and aloe vera gel.
2. Remove from heat and let cool to room temperature.
3. Add essential oil (peppermint, spearmint, Pudinhara) and shake well.
4. Store into an air-tight bottle.

Recipe #3 – Lemon

Ingredients:
1 C Water
1/2 C Plain Soda Drink
4 t Vegetable Glycerin
1 t Aloe Vera Gel
10 drops Lemon Essential Oil

Instructions:
1. Mix all the ingredients in a bottle and shake well.
2. Store in airtight bottle.

Notes:
Never rub pure lemon juice or lemon/lime on your teeth.

Recipe #4 – Tea Tree Oil

Ingredients:
1 C Warm Water
1/2 t Myrrh Tincture
2-4 drops Tea Tree Essential Oil
2-4 drops Peppermint Essential Oil (or spearmint)

Instructions:
1. Mix all the ingredients and gargle.

Nettle Beer for Joint Pain

Treatments:
General joint pain, soreness, inflammation.

Ingredients:
1 lb. Sugar
2 Lemons
1 oz. Cream of Tartar
5 qt. Water
2 lb. Nettle Tops
1 oz. Live Yeast

Instructions:
1. Place sugar, lemon peel (no white), lemon juice, and cream of tartar in a large crock.
2. Cook nettles in water for 15 minutes.
3. Strain into the crock and stir well.
4. When this cools to blood warm, dissolve the yeast in a little water and add to your crock.
5. Cover with several folds of cloth and let brew for three days.
6. Strain out sediment and bottle.
7. Ready to drink in eight days.

Pink Eye

Treatments:
Pink eye, general eye infections.

Ingredients:
1 C Boiling Water
1 t Dried Eyebright Herb

Instructions:
1. Pour the boiling water over the herb.
2. Steep for 10 minutes.
3. Strain and allow to cool.

Dosage:
For pink eye, you can use the liquid one of two ways. You can either use as an eyewash 3-4 times a day –OR– you can use as a warm compress by dipping a soft cloth into the infusion while it's still warm.

If used as a warm compress, then gently wring it out and apply to eyes. Repeat as cloth cools. You may need to reheat your infusion. Leave the compress on the eyes for at least 10 minutes.

Notes:
The herb Eyebright has astringent and antibacterial properties to draw out infections such as pink eye and soothe eyes. You can also purchase eyebright tincture already made from an herbal shop. Put three drops of eyebright tincture in a tablespoon of boiled water. When cool, use as an eyewash.

Respiratory Anthrax (Internal use)

Ingredients:
45 drops Lavender (essential oil)
45 drops Oregano (essential oil)
2 oz. Vodka (or brandy)
10-12 drops Echinacea Tincture
10-12 drops Elderberry tincture
10-12 drops Garlic Tincture
10-12 drops Goldenseal Tincture
1/2 glass of Water

Instructions:
1. Combine all ingredients into the 1/2 glass of water.

Dosage:
Take combined mixture 3 times per day, 10 minutes before meals.

Restless Leg Syndrome

Treatments:
Restless leg.

Ingredients:
1 t Apple Cider Vinegar
1 C Warm Water
Honey (to taste)

Instructions:
1. Add the Apple Cider to the warm water.
2. Add honey to taste (for sweetness).

Dosage:
Once a day regulated (morning or evening).

Rosaleen's Bullwinkle Bars

Ingredients:
4 T Peanut Butter
2 T Honey
2 T Molasses
8 T Oatmeal
1/3 C Powdered Milk
4 T Grits (soy)
4 T Wheatgerm (raw)
3 T Raisins (optional)

Instructions:
1. Combine the peanut butter, honey, and molasses in a bowl then microwave for 60-90 seconds.
   a. When the syrup starts to bubble, remove from microwave regardless of elapsed time.
2. Stir the heated mixture to fully incorporate then add the remaining ingredients.
3. Once thoroughly combined, turn out onto a sheet of wax paper or plastic wrap.
4. Use the wax paper or plastic wrap to form the mixture into a log
5. Slice to desired thickness while warm.

Tip: Depending on the dryness of the weather, and of the ingredients, a little more of the peanut butter or syrup may be needed.

Credit: Rosaleen at Ultralight Joe

Saline Solution

<u>Treatments:</u>
Contact lens cleaner.

<u>Ingredients:</u>
1/4 t Kosher Salt
8 oz. Water
1/4 t Baking Soda

<u>Instructions:</u>
1. Mix all ingredients together.

Sandpiper's Mookies

<u>Ingredients:</u>
8 T Honey
8 T Corn Flour
4 T Peanut Butter
1/4 C Soy Milk Powder

<u>Instructions:</u>
1. Form into balls approximately 1 inch in diameter.
2. Place on unoiled baking sheet and flatten to a 1/4 inch thick with the bottom of a plastic cup dipped gently in corn flour.
   a. Shake off the excess flour. If any is left behind on a Mookie, gently brush it off with a pastry brush.
3. Bake at 350-degrees for 8-10 minutes, or until light golden. Do not overbake!
   a. The easiest way to tell that they're done is to watch when the "sheen" disappears from the surface and it looks dry.
4. Cool on the baking sheet for 5-10 minutes before attempting to move them to a cooling rack. They're very soft when they come out, but do firm up.

Makes a little under two dozen Mookies.

<u>Notes:</u>
For Cherry Mookies, add 3/4 C chopped dried cherries.
For Chocolate Chip Mookies, add 3/4 C mini chocolate chips.

Credit: Sandpiper at Ultralight Joe

Skin Anthrax (Internal use)

Ingredients:
5 drops Cinnamon Bark (essential oil)
8 drops Geranium (essential oil)
5 drops Lavender (essential oil)
5 drops Savory (essential oil)
20 drops Calendula Tincture
20 drops Artichoke Tincture
2 oz. Vodka (or brandy)
1/2 glass of Water

Instructions:
1. Combine all ingredients into the 1/2 glass of water.

Dosage:
Take combined mixture 3 times per day, 10 minutes before meals.

Soap

Recipe #1 – Basic Homemade Soap

Ingredients/Supplies:

2 1/4 C Extra Virgin Olive Oil (can replace EVOO with vegetable oil or animal fat oil (tallow – see Note [1])

1/2 C Coconut Oil (regular coconut oil that melts around 76-degrees F - for moisture)

2 1/2 t Fragrant Essential Oil (can replace with vegetable oil or animal oil)

1/3 C Lye

2/3 C Water (see Note [2])

Soap Molds (see Note [3])

Instructions:

1. In a glass bowl, mix the lye into your water - not the other way around and it is best to do this step outside so that you don't fill your house with the fumes. Try not to breathe the fumes in.
2. Once the lye has dissolved, leave the mix to cool in an area where no kids or pets have access to it.
3. While the lye mixture is cooling, in another glass bowl that has plenty of room to receive the lye mixture and the other remaining ingredients, measure and mix your olive and coconut oils.
4. After the lye mixture has cooled a bit, bring it back inside and pour into your oil mix – mix them together gently at first.
5. Once the lye mixture has been incorporated into your oils, place the bowl in the bottom of your sink and blend them with a hand blender – be careful not to spray the mixture all over. (You can do this step by hand, but it will take a lot longer.)
6. When your mixture starts to thicken like mayonnaise (stage called "trace"), mix in your essential oils – or vegetable oil, or animal fat oil [Note 1].
7. Pour into soap molds [Note 2].
8. Cover and set aside for at least 24 hours – if covered with a cloth (to keep the warmth in), it supposedly contributes to the quality of the soap.
9. After 24 hours, uncover and see if you can unmold it. If it is too soft, wait a few more hours and unmold – try placing it in a cold place to help shrink it a little to aid the unmolding process. Don't wait too long though or it will be too hard to cut into bars.
10. Cut into bars as you see fit.

11. Let the bars dry and harden by letting them sit for around a month – turn every day or two for the first week, and then once a week after that.

Notes:

[1] If you are using pig fat (tallow), please note that it has to be boiled down to separate the oil. Skim off the gunk that floats then strain the oil first.

[2] Once you get the hang of it, you can substitute water with other liquids like coffee to get a nice woodsy coffee smell, or pure strained citrus juice, etc. Use your imagination.

[3] For the molds, you can use silicone soap molds or any other mold you want. However, if it isn't a silicone mold, line the mold with wax paper for easier removal.

Recipe #2 – Soap without Lye

If you want to make bar soap from scratch, without relying on the glycerin melt and pour method, you have to use lye. The melt and pour method is easy and can introduce you to the world of soap making and the fun that you can have with colors and scents. If you choose to try your hand at making soap with lye at a later point, you will already have your scents, colors, and molds all ready to go.

Ingredients/Supplies:
Glycerin block
Sharp knife
Double boiler
Soap dye or colorant
Fragrance
Herbs or other additives
Spoon
Molds

Instructions:
1. Cut the glycerin into 1-inch pieces and place them in the top half of a double boiler.
2. Melt the soap in the top half of the double boiler, stirring occasionally and very gently as it melts.
3. Add in the fragrance and dye one drop at a time until it reaches the color and scent that you desire.
4. Stir in any herbs or additives you wish – stir very gently so as not to introduce bubbles into your soap.
5. Pour your soap mixture into your molds and allow them to cool for at least 2 hours.
6. Remove the soap from the molds – now ready to use.

Recipe #3 – Soap from Plants

There are several plants that are very high in saponins – the substance that makes soap foam and clean. Making plant-based soap is not the same as making soap bars. Instead, this process produces a liquid soap that can be used as hand soap, shampoo, or even a laundry detergent. It is extremely gentle, and good for people that are sensitive to chemicals and additives in other forms of commercial soap. Keep in mind that this form of soap does not last forever; if you choose to make it, do so in small batches and plan on using within a month to keep it fresh.

Ingredients/Supplies:
1/2 C Soapwort Leaves or Roots
4 C Distilled Water
Essential Oil
Tea Tree Oil
Enamel Pan

Instructions:
1. Place the soapwort and distilled water in a large enamel pan.
2. Simmer on low heat for about half an hour, or until suds begin to form in the pan when stirred.
3. Add a few drops of tea tree oil to give it some antibacterial properties, and a few drops of your favorite essential oil to enhance the scent.
4. Allow the mixture to cool and place in an airtight bottle or container until ready to use.

Recipe #4 – Oatmeal Soap

This recipe also uses a 'melt and pour' method by using a type of soap base that can be easily found at most craft stores. The addition of the oatmeal helps make it a great moisturizer for your skin. You can also choose to use goat's milk, honey, or beeswax along with the oatmeal to customize your soap and enhance its skin soothing properties.

Ingredients/Supplies:
8 oz. Clear Soap Base
8 oz. Opaque Soap Base
1/2 oz. Finely Ground Oatmeal
1/2 oz. Essential Oil
1/2 oz. Honey, Beeswax, Goat's Milk, or any other additives
Soap colorant

Instructions:
1. Melt down the two soap bases together and stir very gently to combine.
2. Add any fragrance, colorants, or additives and stir them gently together.
3. Add the oatmeal to the soap mixture. The key is to have the oatmeal ground as finely as possible so it suspends inside the soap and doesn't just settle to the bottom of the bar.
4. Continue to stir very gently until the oatmeal appears to be well distributed throughout the bar.
5. Pour the soap into molds and allow it to harden overnight.
6. Remove from molds and use.

Recipe #5 – Yucca Soap/Shampoo

The yucca plant grows throughout the Midwest and Southwest, but it is mostly found in warmer climates. The roots being edible and the main root of the plant is a tuber, like a potato. When the liquid is pressed out, it can be used as soap or a shampoo. Depending on your location, it is entirely possible that a yucca plant found in the wild is illegal to harvest. Yucca plants on private property are a different matter and generally only require the property owner's permission to harvest. Check you locality laws before trying this recipe.

Ingredient/Supplies:
Yucca plant root (tuber)
Mortar & pestle (Mexican molcajete)

Instructions:
1. Locate a small to medium sized yucca plant.
2. Hold back the thorny ends of the leaves.
3. Use a machete, or long-handled shovel, dig up the plant, tuber root and all.
4. Harvest the main tuber root.
5. Wash and then skin the husk off of the tuber (think pineapple).
6. Dice the tuber into 1/4" to 1/2" size cubes.
7. Grind the tuber cubes as fine as possible. The root is hard and may need to be beaten with the pestle in order to start breaking it down.
8. Once ground, use your hands, and squeeze out any liquid from the ground up root. Any liquid collected can be used for soap or shampoo.
9. The left over ground root can be used to scour dirty dishes and pans if enough pressure is exerted to generate more liquid.

Syrups – Cold, Cough, Flu

Recipe #1 – Amish Cough Syrup

Treatments:
Cough due to cold.

Ingredients:
Lemon Juice
Honey
Castor Oil

Instructions:
1. Mix equal parts of lemon juice, honey, and castor oil.

Dosage:
Adults: 1 T per day.
Children Over 2: 1 t per day.

Recipe #2 – Elderberry Syrup for Flu

Treatments:
Flu prevention and flu-like symptoms.

Ingredients:
7 C Elderberry Juice
8 3/4 C Honey
3 C Vodka (80 proof)

Instructions:
1. Warm the elderberry juice to "hot, but not boiling" temp (between 150-180 degrees).
2. Stir in the honey and stir until it's completely dissolved and blended.
3. Remove from the heat.
4. Stir in the vodka.
5. Pour into sterile jars or bottles (sterilize them by boiling for 5-10 minutes in boiling water, then let drip dry upside down until filling).
6. Cap and label.
7. Store in a cool dark place (or bottle in dark brown glass).

Notes (for Instructions only):
If you're starting with dried berries, put 1 C of berries in a quart jar and pour 2 C of boiling water over top. If they soak it up, add a bit more. Stash in the fridge or a cool, dark place for 24-48 hours. Then strain, and squeeze every bit of liquid you can out by twisting the berries in a muslin towel. You'll need 3 qt. jars to make 7 cups.

Dosage:
Adult prevention: 1 T (15 mls, or 1/2 ounce) 2x a day. If there is active flu in your office or family, double that, or take more often.
Adult Flu Treatment: 1-2 T every 3-4 hours.
Children Treatment (under 12): half the adult dose.
Toddlers and Infants: Talk to your doctor, but generally 1 t at similar intervals to the adult dose should be adequate.

Notes:
You cannot overdose on this so feel free to put it in juice, Jell-O, pour it over ice cream - any way you can get the kids to take it is fine.

Alternative Ingredients #1: If you'd prefer to not use alcohol, try the following as replacement ingredients:

7 C Elderberry Juice

14 C Honey

Then proceed with the instructions noted and ignore the reference to the vodka.

Alternative Ingredients #2: If you don't want to use alcohol AND honey, which is probably a good idea for babies under 1 year old, try the following as replacement ingredients:

7 C Elderberry Juice

11 1/2 C Sugar

Then stir until the sugar is dissolved in the hot juice and bottle.

Recipe #3 – Mild Congestion

Treatments:
Mild congestion of the nasal cavities.

Ingredients:
1 C Tomato Juice
1 t Lemon Juice
1 t Fresh Garlic (minced)
1/2 t Hot Sauce

Instructions:
1. Mix all ingredients in a pan and heat to desired temperature.

Dosage:
Sip until feeling better.

Notes:
You can freeze in ice cube trays for longer term use/storage or just put it the fridge and it will last a few days.

Recipe #4 – Nature's Penicillin

Treatments:
Sore throat, cough.

Ingredients:
24 Cloves Garlic
Raw Honey

Instructions:
1. Peel the garlic and put them in a medium size jar.
2. Add the honey, a little at a time over a couple of days, until the jar is full.
3. Let set it in a sunlit window until garlic has turned somewhat opaque and the honey tastes strongly of garlic.

Dosage:
Take a teaspoon every few hours as necessary.

Recipe #5 – Nighttime Cold Remedy (Nyquil)

Treatments:
Cold and flu.

Ingredients:
1 Lemon
1/4 C Maple Syrup
1/4 C Hot Water
2 T Brandy

Instructions:
1. Squeeze all of the juice from the lemon.
2. Stir the lemon juice into the maple syrup.
3. Add the hot water and brandy.

Dosage:
Drink at once. Repeat after 24 hour, if necessary.

Notes:
This remedy lets you sleep vary soundly all night.

Testicular Discomfort Bath

Treatments:
Testicular soreness and discomfort.

Ingredients:
1 Q Water
1/4 C Comfrey
1/4 C Mullein leaves
1/8 C Chamomile flowers

Instructions:
1. Bring water to a boil and pour it over the herbs
2. Steep at least 15 minutes.
3. Strain and pour into your bath.

Toothpaste

Toothpastes are interesting. Depending on which study you've read, baking soda is either a non-issue or detrimental. Many naturalists and herbalists tend to prefer clay as the primary abrasive because it is so rich in minerals. Clay is good for demineralization and it is highly alkalizing. Therefore, it is a good replacement for baking soda.

White clay is great for general dental use for adults and children. Green clay is slightly more cleansing and toning to the gums. Pink and red clay are soothing. Yellow clay is great for regenerating tissue, as it is very high in natural sulfur, which has a strengthening effect on gum tissue. As a powder, yellow clay can be used straight or mixed into a paste using water, or salt water, or propolis (resinous mixture), or with colloidal silver, or liquid calcium/magnesium etc.

Because of the differing opinions on baking soda, I've provided an assortment of toothpastes and tooth powders.

Recipe #1 – Little Tree Tooth Powder

Ingredients:
2 T White Clay Powder
1-2 t very fine MSM Powder
1 t very fine Xylitol Powder (to taste)
1-5 drops Lemon (or peppermint or fennel essential oils)

Instructions:
1. Combine the ingredients and shake well.
2. Use about 1/4 tsp on a wet toothbrush.

Recipe #2 - Toothpaste for Sensitive Teeth

Ingredients:
1/2 C Vegetable Glycerin
1/2 C Cosmetic Clay (white)
35-40 drops Tincture of Myrrh
7-8 drops Peppermint (or Spearmint or Pudinhara)
7-8 drops Clove Essential Oil

Instructions:
1. Mix all the ingredients thoroughly.
2. Adjust the quantity of glycerin to get toothpaste like consistency.
3. Store in a wide mouth bottle.

Recipe #3 - Tooth Powder

Ingredients:
3 parts Baking Soda
1 part Sea Salt
3 parts Wachter's Cal-Mag-Vit C Powder
3 parts Prickly Ash Bark (finely ground)
1 part Echinacea Powder
1/2 part Goldenseal Powder
Peppermint Essential Oil (to taste)

Instructions:
1. Combine the ingredients and shake well.
2. Use about 1/4 tsp on a wet toothbrush.

Notes:
Most, if not all, of the ingredients are available at a health food store. Recipe does well with tooth sensitivity and gum health.

Recipe #4 – Anti Viral/Bacterial/Fungal Toothpaste

Ingredients:
2 T Coconut Oil
3 T Baking Soda
5 drops Spearmint Essential Oil
Pinch of Stevia powder

Instructions:
1. Mixed ingredients in a tiny wide mouth half-pint canning jar.
2. Dip dry toothbrushes in.

Notes:
Don't get grossed out. Coconut oil is anti-viral, anti-bacterial and anti-fungal, so it will even keep the toothbrushes more sanitary.

Recipe #5 – Dr. Paul Keyes' Toothpaste

Ingredients:
1 part Glycerin
1 part Baking Soda
Capful of Hydrogen Peroxide
Unscented Neutrogena Soap
3-5 drops Wintergreen Oil

Instructions:
1. Add glycerin to baking soda to form a pasty mixture that can be applied to a toothbrush with a spoon or other instrument.
2. Put a capful of hydrogen peroxide in a tumbler.
3. Moisten bristles of toothbrush (multi-tufted) by dipping in peroxide.
4. Rub moistened bristles over cake of unscented Neutrogena soap.
5. Cover bristles with soda-glycerin mixture.
6. While watching in a mirror, brush cheek-sides, and tongue-sides of teeth.
7. Re-dip brush in peroxide as needed.
8. Work mixture between teeth with a flat toothpick or Butler stimulator.

Recipe #6 – Pocket Reduction Toothpaste

Ingredients:
1 part Real Salt (Redmond Utah)
1 part Baking Soda
3% Food Grade Hydrogen Peroxide

Instructions:
1. Mix equal parts Real Salt (Redmond Utah) and baking soda made into a paste using 3% Food Grade Hydrogen Peroxide.

Recipe #7 – Kid Safe Toothpaste

Ingredients:
4 T Coconut Oil
4 T Bentonite Clay
2-3 T filtered water
1/2 t Real Sea Salt
10-15 drops Peppermint Essential Oil
Optional - few drops of liquid sweetener

Instructions:
1. Mix coconut oil, clay, and salt in a small bowl. Start with just one tablespoon of water.
2. Working with the back of a spoon, "cream" the ingredients together and add more water until you like the consistency – add the liquid sweetener here if incorporating
3. Add in the peppermint oil (or cinnamon or spearmint) and then mix until well combined.
4. Store in airtight container.
5. Place a pea-size amount on your toothbrush – safe for kids.

Ultralight Joe's Moose Goo

Ingredients:
2 parts Honey
2 parts Corn Flour (not corn meal)
1 part Peanut Butter

Instructions:
1. Mix ingredients thoroughly.
2. Pack the mixture into Coghlan's squeeze tubes, or cold weather wrap in wax paper.

Notes:
Single squeeze tube proportions (2-3 lunches w/ large tortilla)
8 T Honey
8 T Corn Flour
4 T Peanut Butter

Credit: Ultralight Joe

Water Purification

Ingredients:
Regular Clorox Bleach
Water

Instructions:
- Ratio of Clorox bleach to water for purification:
  o 2 drops bleach per quart of water
  o 8 drops bleach per gallon of water
  o 1/2 t bleach per 5 gallons of water

Tip: if water is cloudy, double the recommended dosages of bleach.

Note:
[1] ONLY use regular Clorox bleach (not fresh scent or lemon) to insure that bleach is at its full strength. [2] Rotate or replace your storage bottle minimally every 3 months.

Withdrawal Symptoms (Smoking/Alcohol/Caffeine)

Treatments:
Withdrawal symptoms related to the quitting of smoking, chewing, dipping, alcohol, or caffeine - does well for nerve pain too.

Ingredients:
1/2 t Valerian Root Tincture
1 t Milky Oat Tincture
1/2 t St. John's Wort Tincture
1/2 t Passionflower Tincture
1/2 t Skullcap Leaves

Instructions:
1. Combine ingredients.

Dosage:
2-5 full droppers a day.

Notes:
If you're a recovering alcoholic, use a glycerite instead of alcohol in your tincture.

Yeast Infection – Tampon Treatment

Treatments:
Vaginal yeast infection

Ingredients:
5 ml Thyme Tincture
5 ml Calendula Tincture
5 drops of Tea Tree Oil (or thyme oil)
1-2 T Water

Instructions:
1. Combine all ingredients and mix.
2. With a tampon still seated in its plastic applicator (plastic wrapper removed), saturate a tampon with this mixture and allow to dry.
3. Use twice daily, once in the morning and once at night for 1 hour at a time.

Dosage:
Twice daily for one hour.

Notes:
[1] Do not reuse a tampon. Make a fresh batch of the mixture each time or double the recipe and saturate 2 tampons at the same time. [2] Drying times vary so sometimes it's best to perform the saturation step the night before and allow for drying overnight.

Chapter 6: Child & Infant Care

The skin is the body's largest organ *and* it has the ability to absorb just about anything it contacts... provided it can fit inside the tiny pore openings. Knowing that, would you rather expose your baby to potentially harmful chemicals or safe and natural ingredients? Most parents would agree that ensuring your baby products are completely natural is worth it. These recipes should help you get started.

Making your own baby products with all natural ingredients is fun to do, it saves money, and most importantly, it ensures that harmful product ingredients do not tax their delicate immune system. Most of the ingredients listed in each recipe can be acquired from your garden or purchased at conventional supermarkets and natural food stores.

Technically, some of these recipes would constitute a salve because they are rubbed on the skin. However, I made an exception and kept all of the recipes specific to children together in one section.

Additionally, because these are recipes specific to infants and younger children, none of the recipes contain alcohol-derived tinctures.

3-C Cream for Children

Treatments:
This cream is especially good for burns or irritated mucous passages, or as a diaper rash ointment.

Ingredients:
1 T Chamomile
1 T Comfrey Root
1 T Marigold Flowers
4 oz. Olive Oil
Dab of beeswax (about 1 T)

Instructions:
1. Mix a thick infusion of the herbs.
2. Strain out the herbs.
3. Add the herbal liquid to the oil.
4. Simmer until most of the water has boiled off.
5. Add the beeswax and heat until it is melted.
6. Remove from the heat and stir until the cream is solid and cooled.

Baby Bath Milk

Treatments:
Skin moisturizer/nourishment.

Ingredients:
1 C Milk
1/4 C Corn Starch
1/4 C Finely Ground Oats
2-3 drops of Lavender, Rose, or Chamomile Essential Oils

Instructions:
1. Mix ingredients together
2. Put in a shaker style bottle.

Dosage:
To use, sprinkle a small amount in warm bath water.

Baby Oil

Treatments:
Skin moisturizer/nourishment.

Ingredients:
1 C Grapeseed Oil (or Apricot Kernel Oil)
4-6 drops Lavender Essential Oil (or Chamomile)
1-2 Vitamin E Capsules (optional)

Instructions:
1. Mix the oils together (or squeeze the vitamin E capsules into the oils and mix together).
2. Store in a dark colored bottle.

Dosage:
Use as a bath or massage oil when necessary.

Baby Wipes

Recipe #1 – Homemade Wipes

Ingredients:
2 C Hot Water, boiled
1 T Baby Bath (or shampoo)
1 T Oil (baby oil, mineral oil, massage oil)
1 T Lotion (baby or regular lotion with/without scent)
1 T White Vinegar (optional but it prevents mold)

Instructions:
1. Mix all ingredients together.
2. Pour over pre-folded paper towels.

Recipe #2 – All Natural Baby Wipes

Treatments:
Use as an anti-fungal, discourages yeast diaper rashes

Ingredients:
1 C Water
1/4 C Aloe Vera Juice
1 T Apple Cider Vinegar
1 T Calendula Oil
1 t Soap (grated, unscented)
2 drops Lavender Oil
2 drops Tea Tree Oil

Instructions:
1. Mix in a jar.
2. Pour over organic cloth wipes or paper towels.

Recipe #3 – Castile Solution

Ingredients:
1 T Almond Oil (can use apricot or other oil)
1 T Dr. Bronner's Pure-Castile Liquid Soap
2 drops Tea Tree Oil
1 drop Lavender Oil
1 C Water

Instructions:
Combine all ingredients in the order noted into a spray bottle and do so very slowly to avoid bubbles.
Use a spray bottle to spritz baby wipes prior to use.

Note:
Mix a new batch every week to avoid mustiness and mildew.

Children's Cough Syrup

Treatments:
Cough due to cold.

Ingredients:
3 Large Onions
1/2-3/4 C Honey
1/2-3/4 C Lemon Juice

Instructions:
1. Peel and slice 3 large onions into a saucepan.
2. Add equal parts honey and lemon juice (start with 1/2 C each).
3. Cook until the onions are translucent then strain.
4. Put the liquid back in the pot and taste it - it should taste about like a honey lemon cough drop with just a hint of onion.

Dosage:
1 T whenever they cough or every hour or so.

Homemade Baby Powder (Talc-Free)

Treatments:
Moisture and wetness reduction.

Ingredients:
1/2 C Corn Starch
1/2 C Arrowroot Powder
1 T Dried Ground Chamomile
1 T Dried Ground Lavender
1/4 C Finely Ground Oats

Instructions:
Blend well and put in a shaker style bottle.

Dosage:
Reapply with diaper change or as necessary.

Homemade Diaper Rash Cure

Treatments:
Diaper rash

Ingredients:
Milk of Magnesia
Corn Starch

Instructions:
1. Mix equal parts milk of magnesia and corn starch together until creamy.
2. Apply liberally to baby.

Homemade Pedialyte

Treatments:
Fluid replacement

Ingredients:
2 qt. Water
1 t Baking Soda
7 T Sugar
1 packet Unsweetened Kool-Aid (any flavor, 1/4 oz.)
1/2 T Salt Substitute

Instructions:
1. Mix all ingredients together really well.
2. Store in the refrigerator for 3 days max.

Dosage:
Provide as needed for fluid replacement during illness.

Notes:
Can be made into ice cubes.

Lavender Dryer Sachets

Treatments:
Baby clothing.

Ingredients:
Dried Lavender
2-3 drops Lavender Essential Oil
1 Muslin Drawstring Bag – small (you can usually get these at craft stores)

Instructions:
1. Fill the muslin bag with dried lavender and add oil.
2. Close the bag tightly and throw in the dryer along with your baby clothes.

Lice Removal Shampoo

Treatments:
Lice

Ingredients:
1 oz. Olive Oil
5 drops Tea Tree Oil
5 drops Rosemary Oil
3 drops Oregano Oil

Instructions:
1. Mix all of the ingredients together.
2. Massage through the child's hair and scalp.
3. Let rest for 10-15 minutes.
4. Rinse thoroughly

Dosage:
Repeat every day for three days or until nits are no longer present.

Natural Hair Detangler

Treatments:
Detangles hair similarly to No More Tangles ™

Ingredients:
8 oz. Distilled Water
1 t Aloe Vera Gel
1-2 drops Glycerin
1-2 drops Essential Oil
15 drops Grapefruit Seed Extract

Instructions:
1. Combine in a spray bottle.
2. Shake before each use.

Peter Rabbit's Tea

Treatments:
Stomach aches, stress, anxiety, nerves and such

Ingredients:
2 C Boiling Water
1 t Chamomile Flowers
1 t Lemon Balm Leaves
1/2 t Catnip Leaves
1/2 t Fennel Seed (or dill seed)

Instructions:
1. Pour boiling water over herbs and steep for 10 minutes.
2. Strain out herbs and allow to cool.
3. Have your child sip this tea as needed, sometimes as little as 1/4 cup spells relief.

Teething Biscuits

Recipe #1 – Dairy Free Vanilla Biscuits

<u>Treatments:</u>
Teething children.

<u>Ingredients:</u>
1 Egg, beaten
1/2 C Sugar
1/2 t Vanilla
1 C Flour

<u>Instructions:</u>
1. Beat the egg then stir in the sugar and vanilla.
2. Add the flour and stir in, until the dough is stiff.
3. Roll out on a lightly floured surface
4. Cut into shapes.
5. Let sit for 12 hours (it's a good idea to make these in the evening then leave the dough overnight).
6. Bake at 350-degrees (176 C) until golden and hard.

Recipe #2 – Dairy Free Italian Biscuits

Treatments:
Teething children.

Ingredients:
2 small Eggs
1 Powdered Sugar
1 C Flour
1/2 t Baking Powder

Instructions:
1. Using an electric mixer, whisk the eggs with the sugar for around 10 mins, until the mixture is thick.
2. Mix the baking powder with the flour, then gradually add the flour to the egg mixture. Increase the amount of flour if the mixture is too sticky.
3. Roll the dough out into long strips, around 1 1/2 in wide, on a lightly floured surface.
4. Place on a baking sheet/cookie sheet.
5. Cover with a clean tea towel and let sit for 12 hrs.
6. Preheat the oven to 375-degrees (190 C).
7. Cut the dough into 1 1/2 in pieces and return to the cookie sheet.
8. Bake 15-20 mins until golden brown.
9. Let cool on wire racks.

Recipe #3 – Cinnamon Cookie Biscuits

Treatments:
Teething children.

Ingredients:
2 1/2 C Flour
1/2 C Non-Fat Dried Milk Powder
1/2 C Wheat Germ
1 1/2 t Baking Powder
1 t Cinnamon
Pinch of Salt
3/4 C Sugar
1/3 C Vegetable Oil
1 Egg, beaten
1/4 C Frozen Apple Juice Concentrate, thawed

Instructions:
1. Mix the flour, milk powder, wheat germ, baking powder, cinnamon and salt in a bowl (dry bowl).
2. Mix the oil and sugar in a separate bowl and beat in the egg (wet bowl).
3. Stir the apple juice into the wet bowl.
4. Begin adding enough of the flour mixture from the dry bowl into the wet bowl to make stiff dough.
5. Place in the refrigerator for 2 hours.
6. Preheat the oven to 375-degrees (190 C)
7. Roll out the dough and cut into shapes, then place on a greased baking sheet/cookie sheet.
8. Bake for 15-20 minutes until golden brown.
9. Let cool on wire racks.

Recipe #4 – Vanilla Biscotti Biscuits

Treatments:
Teething children.

Ingredients:
1/2 C Sugar
1 1/2 T Butter
1 Egg
1/2 t Baking Powder
Pinch of Salt
1 t Vanilla Extract
1 C Flour

Instructions:
1. Preheat the oven to 350-degrees (176 C).
2. Cream the sugar with the butter and beat in the egg.
3. Add the vanilla extract, flour, baking powder and salt and mix the dough well.
4. Form the dough into a long "log" shape and bake for 20 mins on a greased baking sheet/cookie sheet.
5. Allow to cool, then cut into 1/2 in slices.
6. Place each slice, cut side down, on a baking/cookie sheet, then bake for another 15-20 mins, turning the Biscotti over half way through the cooking time.

Recipe #5 – Biscuits with Yeast

Treatments:
Teething Children.

Ingredients:
1 C Milk
1/4 C Tepid Water
1/4 C Butter
1 Egg Yolk, beaten
1 t Salt
4 C Unbleached Flour
2 T Sugar
1 T Active Dry Yeast

Instructions:
1. Place the butter, milk, salt and 1 T sugar in a saucepan. Warm over low heat let cool until tepid.
2. Dissolve the remaining 1 T of sugar with the yeast in the lukewarm water.
3. Cover and set aside.
4. Once bubbling occurs in the yeast mixture, add the milk mixture to the yeast mixture and stir.
5. Add the beaten egg yolk, then gradually add 3 C flour.
6. Mix the dough well continuing to add flour a little at a time to create a soft dough.
7. Turn out and knead the dough on a lightly floured surface until smooth and elastic.
8. Place dough in a greased bowl and cover.
9. Set aside and allow the dough to rise until double in size.
10. Pull off small pieces of dough and, using your hands, roll into small balls.
11. Place on a greased baking sheet/cookie sheet, leaving a few inches between each.
12. Set aside again and allow dough to rise until double in size once more.
13. Bake at 375-degrees (190 C) for 15-20 minutes until golden brown.

Thrush Oil

Treatments:
Oral yeast infection

Ingredients:
8 drops Lavender Essential Oil
8 drops Tree Essential Oil
2 T Vegetable Oil

Instructions:
1. Combine ingredients.
2. Gently apply oil to inside of child's mouth with a cotton swab or a clean finger.

Notes:
A nursing mother whose child is suffering from thrush should apply this oil to her nipples so that she and her baby do not pass the illness back and forth.

Upset Tummy Oil Rub

Treatments:
Stomach aches, colic, gas pains, etc.

Ingredients:
6 drops Lemongrass Essential Oil
1 drop Chamomile Essential Oil
1 drop Fennel Essential Oil
2 oz. Vegetable Oil

Instructions:
1. Mix oils together.

Dosage:
Rub on every hour, or as needed. The recipe also works with lemon balm and can used for children or adults.

Chapter 7: Poultices

Technically, a poultice is a salve covered with a bandage. However, salves tend to be thinner in composition with the consistency fluctuating somewhere between watery and hand cream. A poultice on the other hand, tends to be thicker, like a paste.

Poultice's can be used to treat many things, and have the potential to increase blood flow, relax tense muscles, soothe inflamed tissues, and draw out toxins from an infected area of the body. They are typically used for pain and inflammation caused by things like:

- Abscesses
- Bruises
- Boils
- Fractures
- Pressure ulcers
- Chest congestion
- Remove embedded particulates

Making herbal poultices is not difficult as is noted in the *Basic Herbal Poultice Process* 'recipe'. The 'dried herbs' ingredient in the recipe has been left ambiguous on purpose because different herbs are used for different things based on the inherent properties of the herb.

It is important to note a few things about poultices though. Namely, because a poultice is in direct contact with the skin you should:

- Test a small area on your skin away from the affected area before applying the poultice.
  - Allergic reactions are possible due to direct contact with your skin.
- Use a clean cloth when making a compress for open wounds.
- Never apply a poultice to a wound that appears to be seriously infected.
- Check the temperature of a heated poultice to ensure that you don't burn the skin.

Lastly, you can apply both hot and cold herbal poultices as both of them have their own advantages. A hot poultice improves blood circulation, relieves pain, loosens congestion, and relaxes cramps. A cold poultice is able to decrease inflammation, swelling, fights burns, sprains, bruises, and other kinds of injuries.

Basic Herbal Poultice Process

Ingredients:
1 C Dried Herbs
1 C Boiled Water
Corn Meal, Flour, or French/Bentonite Clay
Flannel or soft cloth

Instructions:
1. Mix the dried herbs with the water.
2. Add enough clay, corn meal, or flour to make a paste thick enough to apply topically.
3. Spread the paste onto a square of cloth that is about 6-8 inches square.
4. Apply the cloth directly to the affected area.

Dosage:
Press the cloth down so the paste sticks to the skin, then cover the area with a dry cloth. Leave the paste on until it dries and pulls away from the skin.

Now that you see how easy it can be to create a poultice, it begs the question. Which herbs and ingredient combinations work best? Chapter 4 is a good place to start. Review the provided ingredients contained there to derive your concoction.

Those herbs notwithstanding, the herb(s) and/or other ingredients chosen for a poultice really depends on what you're treating. For example, the following ingredients can be used in addition to your chosen herbs to make poultices that treat a variety of ailments:

- Activated Charcoal
- Aloe Vera
- Baking Soda
- Bread
- Cat's Claw
- Coconut Oil
- Dandelion
- Epsom salt
- Eucalyptus
- Garlic
- Ginger
- Milk
- Onion
- Turmeric

On the following pages are several poultice recipes that can be used to treat a host of issues associated with an active lifestyle and aging.

Activated Charcoal Poultice

Treatments:
Inflammation caused by a bug bite or sting, or other minor skin irritation.

Ingredients:
1 t Activated Charcoal
Water

Instructions:
1. Combine activated charcoal powder with incremental amounts of water to wet the powder and create a paste.
2. Spread the paste on the affected area.
3. Leave on for 10 minutes.
4. Carefully wash off with a damp cloth.
5. Repeat twice a day until healed.

Aloe Vera Poultice

Treatments:
Scratches, minor skin burns, speed up healing.

Ingredients:
3-4 Plantain Leaves
3-4 Yarrow Leaves
1 Calendula Flower Head
3-4 stalks of Lavender Flower
Aloe Vera Juice

Instructions:
1. Place fresh plant material in a mortar and pestle and crush the herbs until they are a fine mash (like a poultice).
   a. If using dried herbs, place dried material in a blender or spice grinder and break down the material that way, then place in the mortar and pestle.
2. Once the plants are broken down, add Aloe Vera juice to the mix a little at a time, and continue to crush the material with the mortar and pestle.
3. Add more Aloe Vera juice as needed to make it runnier than a typical poultice then cover and let the mixture sit 20 minutes to infuse.
4. Strain the mixture through a fine sieve into a glass spray bottle.
5. Store the spray in the refrigerator. It will keep for about a week.

Dosage:
[1] For sunburns, spray mixture directly on the sunburn. [2] For scratches and minor skin burns, spray on muslin (or gauze) and place on affected area. [3] Do not apply on open, deep wounds.

Notes:
Use witch hazel instead of the Aloe Vera juice for a more shelf stable (longer storage time) version.

Arthritis Poultice

Treatments:
Arthritis and joint pain.

Ingredients:
6 parts Mullein Leaves
9 parts Slippery Elm Bark
3 parts Lobelia
1 part Cayenne
Boiling Water

Instructions:
1. Combine all ingredients except boiling water to create a mixture.
2. Add 3 oz. of the mixture to boiling water to make a paste.

Dosage:
Spread the paste on a cloth and apply to the affected area.

Notes:
Save the remaining mixture of dried ingredients for future use or applications if 3 oz. did not exhaust the mixture.

Ashwagandha Poultice

Treatments:
Joint inflammation.

Ingredients:
Ashwagandha root
Water

Instructions:
1. Crush dried ashwagandha root in a mortar and pestle or gently with a rolling pin or meat tenderizing mallet.
2. Add the crushed root to a bowl and add water incrementally until a thick paste is formed.
3. At the beginning and end of each day, spread the paste on the inflamed joint area and leave in place for 15-30 minutes.

Baking Soda Poultice

Treatments:
Minor skin irritations, such as razor burn or mild sunburn, for a cooling effect.

Ingredients:
2-3 T Baking Soda
Water

Instructions:
1. Combine baking soda with incremental amounts of water to wet the powder and create a paste.
2. Spread the paste on the affected area.
3. Leave on for 10-15 minutes.
4. Carefully wash off with a damp cloth.

Bone Spurs

Recipe #1 – Curcumin and Flaxseed

Treatment:
Bone spurs.

Ingredients:
Curcumin (yellow pigment of turmeric)
Flaxseed

Instructions:
1. Take 500 to 1000 mg of curcumin 3 to 4 times a day on an empty stomach.
2. To relieve pain associated with bone spurs, apply a flaxseed hot pack to the affected area.
3. Take alternate hot and cold footbaths.

Dosage:
Try this remedy daily for about 6 weeks.

Recipe #2 – Linseed Oil

Treatments:
Bone spurs.

Ingredients:
Linseed Oil
Cheese Cloth

Instructions:
1. Warm the linseed oil.
2. Dip a piece of cheesecloth into the warm linseed oil and keep the cloth on the affected area.
3. Cover the cloth with plastic and keep a heating pad on the plastic for 2 hours.

Bran Poultice

Treatments:
Inflammations, strains, sprains, and bruises.

Ingredients:
Bran
Hot Water

Instructions:
1. Make a paste with hot water and bran.
2. Apply as hot as can be tolerated.

Bread Poultice

Treatments:
Thorn or glass removal.

Ingredients:
Wheat Bread
Water

Instructions:
1. Make a paste with hot water and wheat bread.
2. Apply as hot as can be tolerated.

Bread and Milk Poultice

Treatments:
Addresses issues associated with an abscess, cyst, or a splinter.

Ingredients:
2-3 T Milk
Bread Slice

Instructions:
1. Warm the milk in a small pan on low heat.
2. Turn off the stove, remove the pan from heat, and let it cool so it's warm to the touch (not too hot).
3. Place the slice of bread in the pan and let it soften in the milk.
4. Stir the milk and bread to breakdown the bread and make a paste.

Dosage:
Apply the paste to the skin and leave on for 15 minutes. Repeat two or three times a day.

Cabbage Poultice

Treatments:
Ulcers, varicose veins, shingles, eczema, gout, rheumatism, and infection.

Ingredients:
Cabbage (raw or cooked)

Instructions:
1. Place whole leaves layered over area and covered with a hot towel.

Notes:
When applied to lower abdomen: promotes pelvic circulation and dissolves small fibroids and cysts. When applied to liver: breaks up congestion and detoxifies (use for 10 minutes then add more time after multiple applications as it can cause a strong detoxification reaction).

Carrot Poultice

Treatments:
Cysts, tumors, boils, cold sores, and skin infections (impetigo).

Ingredients:
Carrots
Vegetable Oil

Instructions:
1. Boil carrots until soft or use raw and mash to a pulp.
2. Mix with small amount of vegetable oil.
3. Apply to infected area.

Cat's Claw Poultice

Treatments:
Inflammation and infections.

Ingredients:
2-3 T Cat's Claw (bark and/or root)
Water

Instructions:
1. Add cat's claw to a mortar and pestle and grind.
2. Add water to make a paste.
3. Smear paste on muslin, cotton cloth, or gauze and apply to the affected area.

Clay Poultice

Treatments:
Inflammatory skin diseases, bruises, sprains, acne, and for drawing toxins from the skin.

Ingredients:
Clay (free of impurities)
Water or Apple Cider Vinegar

Instructions:
1. Mix clay with water or apple cider vinegar to make a paste.
2. Apply to infected area and allow it to dry before removing with warm water.

Coconut Oil Poultice

Treatments:
Helps cuts and scrapes heal quickly.

Ingredients:
1-2 T Yellow clay
Coconut oil

Instructions:
1. Combine clay with enough oil to make a paste.
2. Apply to muslin and place on affected area.

Dandelion Poultice

Treatments:
Acne, eczema, itching, psoriasis, rashes, abscesses, and boils.

Ingredients:
Dandelion Root
Warm Water

Instructions:
1. Crush or process dandelion root into a powder.
2. Add warm water to make a thick paste
3. Apply to muslin and place on affected area.

Epsom Salt Poultice

Treatments:
Abscesses (boils).

Ingredients:
Epsom salt
Warm Water

Instructions:
1. Dissolve Epsom salt in warm water.
2. Soak a compress in the solution.

Dosage:
Apply the compress to the affected area three times a day for twenty minutes.

Eucalyptus Poultice

Treatments:
Chest congestion.

Ingredients:
10 Eucalyptus Leaves
15 Myrtle Leaves

Instructions:
1. Combine and crush ingredients in a mortar and pestle.
2. Place poultice paste on muslin and tie off.
3. Soak in simmering water until warm.
4. Place muslin bag on chest and breathe deeply.

Notes:
Can be re-heated and re-applied until fragrance is lost.

Garlic Poultice

Treatments:
Illness (cold and flu when wheezing and/or coughing is present), external wounds, and ear infections.

Ingredients:
2-3 Garlic Cloves
Warm Water

Instructions:
1. Crush the garlic so it is nice and juicy (a garlic press or fork works well).
2. Place the crushed garlic in cheesecloth then fold into a pocket.
3. Place poultice into a bowl of warm water for a few seconds then squeeze out the excess water.

Dosage:
1. Rub olive oil or petroleum jelly on the skin to protect against skin irritation, then apply poultice to affected area two minutes at a time.
2. Allow skin to rest before re-applying.

Ginger Poultice

See Herbal Poultice.

Herbal Compress for Bleeding

Treatments:
General bleeding and slow healing wounds.

Ingredients:
1 t Tincture of Yarrow
1/2 C Water
Soft cloth

Instructions:
1. Combine ingredients.
2. Soak the cloth in the liquid.
3. Wring it out.
4. Apply it with pressure over the wound.

Notes:
Change bandaging as necessary.

Herbal Poultice

Treatments:
Relieves minor inflammation, abrasions, and more.

Ingredients:
1 t Turmeric Powder
1 oz. Ginger (freshly chopped or grated)
1/4 Small Onion (raw and sliced)
1 Garlic Clove (chopped)
2 t Coconut Oil
Cheesecloth (or cotton bandage)

Instructions:
1. Add the coconut oil followed by the rest of the ingredients to a pan on low heat and allow it to heat until it's almost dry — but not burnt.
2. Turn off the stove and transfer the ingredients to a bowl to cool until it is only warm to the touch.
3. Lay the cloth flat and add the mixture to the center of the cloth.
4. Fold the cloth over twice to create a pack or gather it and tie with some string or a rubber band to create a handle (whatever you prefer as long as the ingredients stay inside the cloth).

Dosage:
Place on the affected area for 20 minutes.

Mustard Poultice

Treatments:

Arthritic joints and any condition requiring increased circulation. Also relieves cough and congestion, aids asthma, and assists in getting rid of colds and flu when used on the chest.

Ingredients:
Powdered Mustard
Water
Flour (optional)

Instructions:
DO NOT APPLY DIRECTLY TO THE SKIN!
1. Mix powdered mustard and water to make a paste (may need to add flour to hold the paste together).
2. Wrap the area in muslin or cheesecloth or a cotton towel so there is a layer between the skin and poultice.
3. Apply the poultice to the added layer.
4. Cover with plastic wrap - remove immediately if stinging or burning occurs.

Notes:
Use with caution. Do not use on sensitive or broken skin.

Onion Poultice

Treatments:

Draws out impurities. High sulfur content makes it good for inflamed areas. Also good for congestion and unproductive coughs and ear infections.

Ingredients:
Onion (chopped)
1-2 T Flour
Olive Oil (or vegetable)

Instructions:
1. Sautee chopped onion in oil and flour.
2. Wrap in cheesecloth and apply to area.

Plantain Poultice

Treatments:
Burns, cuts, scrapes, insect bites, reduce inflammation, prevent infection, and speed healing.

Ingredients:
1/4-1/2 C Boiling Water
1/2 C Plantain Leaves (dried or fresh)

Instructions:
1. Place a 1/4 C of boiling water in a blender and add the plantain leaves.
2. Blend on slow speed.
3. Add more water as needed slowly to make a non-watery paste.
4. Spread over the affected area, cover with sterile gauze, and secure in place.

Potato Poultice

Treatments:
Reduce arthritic inflammation and address boils and abscesses.

Ingredients:
Potato (raw)
Boiling Water

Instructions:
1. Grate the raw potato.
2. Mix with boiling water.
3. Apply to affected area.

Turmeric Poultice

Treatments:
Aches, pains, sprains, anti-inflammatory, and pain relief.

Ingredients:
1 T Turmeric Powder
1 T Himalayan Salt
2 T Castor Oil (can use sesame or olive oil)
2-3 T Flour
Water

Instructions:
1. In a stainless steel saucepan, measure out the turmeric, castor oil and salt, then mix to combine.
2. Add the first tablespoon of flour.
3. Add more flour a tablespoon at a time and stop when the mixture comes together in as a thick paste.
4. Warm the mixture on a low flame - splash a few drops of water in the pan to prevent the turmeric from sticking or burning.
5. When it's done it will come together.
6. Allow the poultice to cool (still warm though) and then spread on 1/2 of the cotton flannel.
7. Now apply the poultice to the treatment area and cover by winding the rest of the flannel around if possible and then securing with a safety pin. As an extra precaution, wrap with plastic wrap.

Dosage:
- Rest the area for as long as possible, 30-45 minutes at a minimum (preferably for at least 2-3 hours).
- Apply additional heat by placing a warm water bottle over the treated area.
- The treatment may be repeated 2-3 times a day or left on overnight.

Notes:
[1] This poultice stains the skin but this disappears in 2-3 days. [2] The same poultice can be re-used, just reheat it in a pan, and add a little more castor oil if it is dry.

Chapter 8: Salves

Below are some general tips for making a good salve.

1. Make sure you label your jars!
2. Cold pressed virgin olive oil is best for medicinal salves but if you wish to make a massage salve, you can use a lighter oil such as organic grapeseed oil or almond oil.
3. For massage or perfume salves, only add about 1/4 teaspoon of a floral essential oil to the salve recipe. Rose, lavender, or jasmine would be sensual.
4. To clean the wax out of your pan, fill it with water and bring to a hard boil then dump it out quickly!

Aches and Pains - Camphorated Oil Liniment

Treatments:

Addresses minor aches and pains, sprains, bruises, rheumatic or gouty problems of the joints, and other local pain or glandular swellings.

Ingredients:
1 oz. Camphor USP
4 fl. oz. Olive Oil

Instructions:
1. Dissolve the camphor in the oil.

Notes:

Check skin for sensitivity/allergens to camphor before full use of this liniment. Also, if camphor is available, consider using rosemary as the oil in these leaves contains 10%-20% camphor.

Antibacterial Powder

Treatments:

Prevent and treat general infections, parasitic infections (such as ringworm or mange), or hair loss on pets and animals.

Ingredients:
1 part Golden Seal Powder
1 part Garlic Powder

Instructions:
1. Mix ingredients together and store in a covered jar.

Dosage:
Apply freely to any sore or abraded area where bacteria might become a problem.

Anti-Fungal

Ingredients:
2 parts Chaparral
2 parts Black Walnut Hulls
1 part Golden Seal
1 part Myrrh
1 part Echinacea
Olive Oil (or Tea Tree Oil)
Beeswax
Cajeput Essential Oil

Instructions:
1. Combine all the "part" ingredients in a glass jar.
2. Add a few drops of the Cajeput Essential Oil (or tea tree oil).
3. Fill remaining space in the jar with Olive Oil.
4. Set the jar in the sun for 2 weeks.
5. After 2 weeks in the sun, strain the oil then measure the amount of captured oil.
6. For every cup of oil captured, add 1/4 C Beeswax.
7. Bottle up, seal, and store.

Notes:
For a harder salve, add more beeswax. For a softer salve, add less. Salve will store for years if in a cool, dark place.

Anti-Herpes Paste

Treatments:
Herpes, genital sores.

Ingredients:
1 part Goldenseal Powder
1 part Black Walnut Hull Powder
1 part Echinacea Root Powder
St. John's Wort / Calendula tincture

Instructions:
1. Mix the powder herbs together.
2. Moisten the mixture with a bit of St. John's Wort / Calendula tincture to make a paste.

Dosage:
Apply directly to the sores.

Astringent Liniment

Treatments:
Aches and pains

Ingredients:
1 part Yarrow
1 part Shepherd's Purse
1 part Calendula
1/4 part Cayenne

Instructions:
1. Mix the herbs then cover with warmed vinegar and / or witch hazel extract.
2. Let the mixture sit for 2 to 3 week.
3. Strain in a cheesecloth lined strainer and rebottle.

Notes:
This liniment will last indefinitely and can be used as an astringent for muscular pain and aches.

Black Ointment (aka Ichthyol, Ichthammol, or Drawing Salve)

Treatments:
Sebaceous cysts, boils, ingrown toenails, and splinters.

Ingredients:
3 T Comfrey, Calendula, and Plantain Infused Olive Oil [1]
2 t Shea Butter
2 T Coconut Oil
2 T Beeswax
1 t Vitamin E Oil
2 T Activated Charcoal Powder
2 T Kaolin Clay
1 T Honey
20 drops Lavender Essential Oil

Instructions:
1. Combine all ingredients.
2. Apply liberally and rub into area.
3. Store in an airtight container.

Dosage:
Clean and re-apply as necessary.

Notes:
[1] The olive oil is infused with all three ingredients.
[2] The black ointment salve is also known as 'Ichthyol Salve', 'Ichthammol Ointment', and the 'Drawing Salve'.

Bursitis

Treatments:
Inflammation associated with bursitis.

Ingredients:
3 drops Rosemary
3 drops Geranium
3 drops Eucalyptus
1 T carrier Oil (olive, coconut, rosehip, etc.)

Instructions:
Mix ingredients and rub gently into the area.

Calendula Comfrey Salve

Treatments:
All purpose salve.

Ingredients:
1 C of Olive Oil, cold pressed
1/2 oz. Calendula (dried)
1/2 oz. Comfrey (dried)
1/2 oz. Beeswax (grated)
3 Vitamin E Capsules (at least 400 units - this is your preservative)
Cheesecloth to strain herbs

Tip: You can use 1/2 t of liquid Vitamin E if you have it instead of the three capsules.

Instructions:
1. Place your herbs into an oven safe dish (not aluminum), then add olive oil.
2. Stir and bake in the oven at the lowest possible temperature (200 degrees or less) and bake for 3 hours.
3. Allow the mix to cool slightly, then strain through the cheesecloth-lined strainer while still warm. Squeeze out all the oil you can.
4. Place mixture in a pot on the stove (double boiler preferred) and very gently heat the oil mix back up. Be careful not to burn the mixture.
5. Add the Vitamin E (if capsule, you need to open/separate/puncture the capsules and empty the contents – do not add the actual capsule) and beeswax.
6. Stir until completely melted and blended.
7. Remove from heat and let cool for a minute or two then pour into a wide mouth jar or several small jars. As it cools the mixture will become semi-solid and the perfect salve consistency.

Cold and Flu - Lung Fever

Ingredients:
12oz Unsalted Lard
2 oz. Camphor
3 oz. Beeswax
3 oz. Rosin (powdered)
2 t Raw Linseed Oil
20 ml Turpentine

Instructions:
1. Heat the salt, lard, camphor, beeswax, and rosin in a double boiler.
2. Remove from heat, then add the linseed oil and turpentine.
3. Let cool then bottle as it will store for years.

Treatments:
Used for colds and pneumonia, rub on chest and back.

Comfrey Gel

Treatments:
Burns and abrasions.

Ingredients:
1 C Comfrey Root (fresh chopped)
1 C Water

Instructions:
1. Combine ingredients and simmer for 20 minutes over medium to low heat.
2. Let the mixture cool, then strain through a coarse sieve.

Dosage:
Rub gel onto injured area on a regular basis until condition improves.

Notes:
You can use the resulting gel immediately or roll in to small balls and freeze for future use.

Garlic Oil

Treatments:
Antibacterial, antiviral, and antifungal.

Ingredients:
6 Garlic Cloves
2 T olive oil

Instructions:
1. Crush or squeeze six cloves of garlic into a cup.
2. Add 2 tablespoons olive oil.
3. Allow the active ingredient in the garlic to seep into the oil for three days.
4. Strain off the garlic residue and apply the oil with a cotton swab or cotton ball once daily for a week. If irritation occurs, stop use immediately.

Genital Infection/Irritation

Treatments:
Genital infections and irritations.

Ingredients:
1/8 t Lavender
1/8 t Tea Tree Essential Oils
1 oz. Vegetable Oil

Instructions:
1. Combine ingredients.
2. Apply to the infected or irritated area.

Dosage:
At least 2 times a day.

Notes:
Works well even when the irritation is not caused by infection.

Homemade Neosporin

Treatments:
Similar to the "Plantain Ointment," this can be used on bites, stings, cuts, poison ivy, diaper rash, or other wounds.

Ingredients:
2 C Olive Oil (or Almond Oil)
1/4 C Beeswax Pastilles
1 t Echinacea Root (optional)
2 T Dried Comfrey Leaf
2 T Dried Plantain Leaf (herb not banana)
1 T Dried Calendula Flowers (optional)
1 t Dried Yarrow Flowers (optional)
1 t Dried Rosemary Leaf (optional)

Instructions:
1. Infuse the herbs into the olive oil. (This can be accomplished two ways. Either combine the herbs and the olive oil in a jar with an airtight lid and leave for 3-4 weeks, shaking daily OR heat the herbs and olive oil over low/low heat in a double boiler for 3 hours until the oil is very green.)
2. Strain the herbs out of the oil by pouring through cheesecloth.
3. Let all the oil drip out and then squeeze the herbs to get the remaining oil out.
4. Discard the herbs.
5. Heat the infused oil in a double boiler with the beeswax until melted and mixed.
6. Pour into small tins, glass jars or lip chap tubes and use on bites, stings, cuts, poison ivy, diaper rash or other wounds as needed.

Plantain Lotion

Treatments:
Weeping and itchy rashes, and insect bites.

Ingredients:
Plantain Leaves (finely chopped)
Glycerin

Instructions:
1. Fill a small jar with chopped plantain leaves.
2. Cover leaves with glycerin.
3. Let stand for two weeks, stirring from time to time.
4. Strain and store in dark bottle.

Dosage:
Apply to affected area as needed.

Plantain Ointment

Treatments:
Diaper rash, insect bites, all itches, and minor wounds.

Ingredients:
Plantain Leaves
Olive Oil
Beeswax

Instructions:
1. Pick plantain leaves when they are vibrant and green.
2. Chop them coarsely and pack loosely into a clean, very dry jar.
3. Add olive oil, dislodge air bubbles with a knife or chopstick until the jar is filled to the very top.
4. Label and cap securely.
5. Let sit out of direct sunlight, on a surface that won't be marred by oozing oil.
6. Decant after six weeks, pouring off the oil and squeezing out what remains in the plant material.
7. Discard the herb.
8. Grate 1 T of beeswax for every ounce of oil.
9. Stirring constantly, heat the oil and beeswax until the wax melts, usually within a minute.
10. Pour the liquid into small, wide-mouthed jars and cool.

Dosage:
Use liberally when needed.

St. John's Wort Salve

Treatments:
Aches, pains, bumps, and bruises

Ingredients:
4 oz. St. John's Wort Oil
1/2 oz. Beeswax
Vitamin E (preservative)

Instructions:
1. Place the St. John's Wort Oil and beeswax, along with a few drops of Vitamin E, into a small crock-pot.
2. Set the crock to low and stir occasionally until the beeswax is melted.
3. While warm, pour into a jar, let it set, and then seal the jar.

Dosage:
Apply a thin layer to affected area.

Notes:
Do not use on open wounds.

Tiger Balm

Treatments:
General soreness, aches, and pains.

Ingredients:
1 oz. Cayenne Infused Oil
3 oz. Goldenrod (or Arnica) Infused Oil
3/4 oz. Beeswax
20 drops White Camphor Essential Oil
20 drops Cinnamon Leaf Essential Oil
20 drops Rosemary Essential Oil
30 drops Clary Sage Essential Oil
10 drops Sweet Birch Essential Oil

Instructions:
1. Melt beeswax, add infused oils and stir well.
2. Let cool for a bit before adding essential oils.
3. Mix well and pour into clean, sterilized container.

Notes:
Be careful not to use near body orifices or on open skin.

Vapor Rub

Treatments:
Congestion.

Ingredients:
1/4 t Eucalyptus (essential oil)
1/8 t Peppermint (essential oil)
1/8 t Thyme (essential oil)
1/4 C Olive Oil

Instructions:
1. Combine ingredients in a glass bottle.
2. Shake well to mix oils evenly.
3. Gently massage into chest and throat.

Vinegar of Four Thieves

Treatments:

General cleanser for floors, walls, windows and will offset smells in the home. Deter bugs if you rinse your hiking gear in it. Repurpose the herbs after straining and place were ants come in. Contains antifungal, antibacterial, and antiviral properties.

Ingredients:
2 quarts Apple Cider Vinegar
2 T Lavender
2 T Sage
2 T Rue
2 T Rosemary
2 T Wormwood
2 T Mint
2 T Garlic
4 oz. Glycerin

Instructions:
1. Combine the herbs and steep in vinegar in the sun for 2 weeks.
2. Strain then add 2 tablespoons of garlic buds
3. Steep for several days.
4. Strain in a cheesecloth-lined strainer.
5. To preserve, add 4 oz. of glycerin.

Yarrow Skin Wash

Treatments:
Soothes chapping and minor irritations.

Ingredients:
2 C Boiling Water
1 C Crumpled Dried Flowering Yarrow Tops

Instructions:
1. Pour boiling water over yarrow tops.
2. Let cool, and strain.
3. Pat on the skin.

Notes:
Yarrow makes an excellent skin wash, particularly beneficial to oily complexions. See *Tincture of Yarrow* in Chapter 9: Tinctures.

Chapter 9: Tinctures

A tincture is an herbal remedy made by soaking selected herbs (or parts of herbal plants) in alcohol. The creation of a tincture can take anywhere from two to six or even eight weeks depending on the ingredients and the desired level of potency. It is important to note that the alcohol works as a solvent that allows the healthy benefits of the ingredients to be extruded from the plant material into the alcohol.

Just about any herb can be preserved as a tincture. The key is gathering the medicinal knowledge and understanding with regard to specific healthy/healing properties that are being extracted from each herb or combination of herbs.

The following is a generalized tincture procedure:

Generalized Tincture Procedure:

In a quart size glass jar (Mason), add:

- Enough flower/stem/root ingredients to fill the jar at least half-way.
- Add enough vodka (or rum depending) to cover the ingredients plus 2" above.
- Fill the remaining space in the jar with distilled water.
- Seal jar with an airtight lid and wait 2 to 8 weeks (duration and agitation are dependent on the tincture)

NOTE: Some tincture recipes will call for boiling water instead of distilled water.

Additionally, given the Generalized Tincture Procedure noted above, it is important to point out that some recipes will swap the alcohol and water ingredients. Meaning, depending on the recipe, it may call for the herbs to be submerged in water (boiling or distilled) first, and then fill the remaining space with the specified alcohol. So be sure to read the entire recipe before beginning.

The herb/root ingredients that you choose to add *are* what adds the healing properties and the medicinal qualities to the tincture. Making a tincture is the most cost effective way to use and preserve medicinal herbs.

> **It is incredibly important to note that pregnant women, those that are nursing, or those with a medical condition should check with your doctor or midwife before using any herbal remedy or supplement.**

Now that you know *how* to make a tincture, let's discuss *why* you should potentially make your own. A homemade tincture is:

- More powerful and lasts longer than dried herbs
- Less expensive than buying ready-made herbal products
    o You can make about a quart of your own tincture for the price of a few ounces of tincture at retail stores
- Higher quality due to personally sourced natural ingredients
- Higher purity than store bought remedies
- Customizable
    o Special combination formulas can be derived based on preferences and common familial symptoms
- Mentally rewarding
    o There is something to be said about getting involved in your own health. Some herbalists say that you benefit by absorbing some of the herb through the skin and from the aroma.

How to Make Your Own Tinctures

Materials:

Wide-mouthed glass jars with lids (Mason jar or equivalent).
Unbleached cheesecloth or muslin.
Labels and markers.

Ingredients:

Dried or fresh herbs in powdered or cut form.
80-100 proof vodka or rum (NEVER use rubbing, isopropyl, or wood alcohol).

Instructions:

Many herbalists suggest that you should plan to start your tinctures on the day of the new moon and let them sit at least 2 weeks until the full moon. It is said that this adds a natural drawing power.

1. Pour the amount of herb you desire into the glass jar
2. Slowly pour the alcohol until the herbs are entirely covered.
3. Add distilled water to fill the remainder of the jar.
4. Seal the jar tightly so that the liquid cannot leak or evaporate.
5. Place the jar in a dark area or inside a paper bag.
6. Shake the jar every day.
7. When ready to bottle, pour the tincture through a cheesecloth into another jar or dark colored tincture bottle(s).
8. Squeeze the saturated herbs, extracting the remaining liquid until they stop dripping.
9. Close the storage container with a stopper or cap and label.

Notes:

[1] Generally, measure ~14 tablespoons dried or ~20 tablespoons of fresh herbs (chopped) to one liter of liquid. [2] Incorporate rum to help hide the taste of bitter herbs. **[3] Use distilled water, vinegar, or glycerol to make nonalcoholic tinctures.** [4] The standard dosage is 1 teaspoon, 1-3 times daily, diluted in tea, juice, or water. [5] A tincture can last up to two years when stored in a tightly closed container. [6] A wine press or juicer can be used to extract essential oils from herbs. [7] Several herbs can be combined into a tincture formula.

Now that you've read about tincture basics, here are some tincture recipes for you to try out. Tinker with the recipes to make them your own and tailor them to your needs.

Antidepressant

Ingredients:
1 t St. John's Wort Tincture
1/2 t Licorice Root Tincture
1/2 t Ginseng Root Tincture
1/2 t Lemon Balm Leaf Tincture
1/2 t Ashwaganda Leaf Tincture (if available)

Instructions:
1. Combine ingredients

Dosage:
1 dropperful 3 times a day

Notes:
[1] If you do not, or cannot, drink alcohol, buy/use glycerites instead of tinctures containing alcohol.

Anti-Inflammatory Turmeric and Pepper Tincture

Treatments:
Chronic inflammation and pain from arthritis.

Ingredients:
3 T Turmeric (ground)
5 T Olive Oil (or walnut oil if no allergies*)
3/4 t Black Pepper (finely ground)
1 t Ginger (ground) - optional

Instructions:
1. Add all ingredients (ginger optional) to a small glass container (jelly jar) and mix well.
2. Mix well before each dose.

Dosage:
1 t each morning before breakfast.

Notes:
Walnut Oil contains Omega 3 fatty acids which has anti-inflammatory properties.

Artichoke Bitters Tincture

<u>Treatments:</u>
Digestion.

<u>Ingredients:</u>
1 T Artichoke Leaf
1 T Orange Peel
1 T Cardamom Pods
Vodka

<u>Instructions:</u>
1. Place each ingredient in their own jelly jar.
2. Cover each ingredient vodka (equal amount in each jar).
3. Seal and let the jars sit for one week, shaking gently once a day.
4. Strain each jar through a cheesecloth-lined strainer.
5. Combine equal parts into a tincture bottle(s).

<u>Dosage:</u>
2 dropperfuls in 8 oz. of water (or club soda) 15-20 minutes before a meal.

Artichoke Tincture

Treatments:
Digestion.

Ingredients
1/4 C Hawthorn Berries
1/4 C Dandelion Root
1 T Fennel Seed
1 t Black Pepper (fresh ground)
1/4 C Hibiscus (whole)
1 T Artichoke Leaves
2 T Coriander Seeds
1 Orange (diced, include the peel and seeds)
1/3 C Honey
Vodka

Instructions
1. Place all the herbs, spices, and orange into a quart-sized Mason jar.
2. Add the honey, then fill the jar with the vodka. Stir well.
3. Cover with a lid and shake once or twice a day.
4. Taste after 1 week. If the flavor is acceptable, strain in a cheesecloth-lined strainer. If not, continue to infuse for an additional week.
5. Store in a dark bottle or dark location.

Dosage:
1/2 t in a small amount of water 15 minutes before you eat.

Ashwagandha Leaf Tincture

Treatments:
Stress, anxiety, depression, boost brain function, lowers blood sugar and cortisol levels.

Ingredients:
2 C Ashwagandha Leaves
Vodka

Instructions:
1. Roughly chop the ashwagandha leaves and loosely pack a pint-size mason jar.
2. Fill the jar with vodka.
3. Use a wooden spoon to push down any floaters and remove most of the bubbles.
4. Store in a cool dark place for four to six weeks, shake gently on occasion.
5. Strain through a fine mesh cloth into a clean largemouth jar and squeeze out as much liquid as possible.
6. Pour the liquid via funnel into tincture bottles and store in a cool, dark area.

Dosage:
1/4 t three times a day.

Bay Leaf

Treatments:

Coughs, colds, bronchitis, chest infections, aches, pains, headaches, sprains, swelling, rheumatic, and arthritic pain. New research suggests that a Bay Leaf Tincture can reduce the risk of cardiovascular diseases and Types 2 Diabetes.

Ingredients:

6 oz. Bay Leaves (dried)

1 1/2 - 1 3/4 C Vodka or Rum (enough to cover Bay Leaf)

1 1/2 - 1 3/4 C Boiling Water (enough to fill the rest of the jar)

Instructions:

1. Add the bay leaves to wide mouth 1 qt. jar.
2. Cover the bay leaves with the vodka.
3. Fill the rest of the jar with water.
4. Seal with an airtight lid and store in cool dark spot, shake once a day for 2 weeks to 1 month.
5. Strain and save the liquid.

Dosage:

Soak a cloth with the tincture and then apply and rub/massage the affected area.

Notes:

This recipe is NOT FOR PREGNANT WOMEN.

Black Walnut Tincture

Treatments:
Intestinal parasites, intestinal discomfort/issues, assorted skin conditions, and athlete's foot. See the Notes section for additional uses.

Ingredients:
6-7 Black Walnuts (Fresh, green, whole, and still in the hull)
80 Proof Vodka
1/4 C Olive Oil
2T Lemon Juice

Materials:
Quart canning jar with lid
Gloves
One small dark-colored glass bottle (with dropper)
Sharp Knife

Instructions:
1. Fill a quart canning jar about 2/3 full with vodka.
2. Cut the walnut hulls and place the hulls in the jar.
3. Pour about 2 tablespoons of lemon juice in to help preserve the tincture.
4. Pour about 1/4 cup of olive oil in to help create a barrier from oxidation over time.
5. Make sure the top of the hulls are covered with the vodka, lemon juice, and olive oil mix.
6. Cap the filled jar, without stirring the mix, then place in the refrigerator.
7. Once the tincture is ready to use, strain the mix to remove the hulls and excess debris.
8. Pour the liquid into small dark colored bottles that have droppers.

Dosage:

For intestinal issues, drop 20 small drops of the tincture into a glass of water and drink three times a day until you are feeling better.

For athlete's foots, add one dropperful of the tincture into a gallon of warm water in a small tub, and use as a foot soak.

Notes:

[1] One 2 oz. bottle contains approximately 60 doses.

[2] For topical skin conditions, dip a cotton swab in the tincture and dab on the area in question.

[3] This will stain your skin, and anything else, for a while. However, in its diluted state, staining is less likely to occur on the skin for long periods.

[4] In addition to fending off and preventing various infections and intestinal parasites, other uses include:

- Reducing excessive sweating
- Lowering cholesterol and blood pressure levels
- Aiding in digestion
- Slowing down heavy menstrual bleeding
- Relieving heartburn, colic, diarrhea, and flatulence
- Balances blood sugar levels
- Battles heart disease
- Helps with skin conditions such as acne, boils, and warts

Blue Vervain Tincture

Treatments:
Nervous system, emotional and psychological well-being, anxiety, feeling of being overwhelmed.

Ingredients:
Blue Vervain Flowers and Leaves (no stalks)
Vodka

Instructions:
1. Harvest the Blue Vervain and remove all leaves and flowers from the stalk. Discard the stalks.
2. Roughly chop the harvested material and fill a pint sized Mason jar.
3. Pour vodka into the jar and use a wooden spoon to remove gaps and air bubbles.
4. Store in a dark place away from sunlight and let steep for 4-6 weeks.
5. Shake occasionally.
6. Strain through a fine mesh cloth into a clean largemouth jar and squeeze out as much liquid as possible.
7. Pour the liquid via funnel into tincture bottles and store in a cool, dark area.

Dosage:
1/2 to 1 dropperfuls in water or tea if not treating anxiety. For anxiety treatments, 1 to 2 dropperfuls in water or tea.

Bupleurum Root Tincture

Treatments:

Respiratory infections, influenza, swine flu, common cold, bronchitis, and pneumonia.

Ingredients:

Bupleurum root
Vodka

Instructions:

1. Fill a pint size Mason jar 1/2 full with Bupleurum root.
2. Add enough vodka to cover the root by at least an inch.
3. Store in a cool dark place for four to six weeks, shake gently on occasion.
4. Strain the liquid and squeeze out as much liquid as possible.
5. Pour the liquid via funnel into tincture bottles and store in a cool, dark area.

Dosage:

1/2 to 1 t as needed.

Calendula Tincture

Treatments:

Sore throat and mouth, menstrual cramps, cancer, and stomach and duodenal ulcers. Has also been historically used for measles, smallpox, and jaundice. Can be applied to the skin to reduce pain and swelling (inflammation) and to treat poorly healing wounds and leg ulcers.

Ingredients:
1/2 C Dried Calendula Petals
1 C 80-proof Vodka

Instructions:
1. Add 1/2 C of dried calendula petals to a clean pint sized Mason jar.
2. Cover the dried flowers with 1 C of vodka (use twice as much alcohol as calendula).
3. Seal the jar but do NOT place in the sunlight.
4. Let the concoction steep for 2-8 weeks.
5. Strain the mixture and transfer to tincture bottles.
6. Label and store in cool dark place.

Cayenne Tincture

Treatments:

See Chapter 10: Additional Information, Cayenne: A Remarkable Healing Herb for more information on cayenne.

Ingredients:

Cayenne Peppers (or Habanero)
Vodka

Instructions:

1. Wash and dry all peppers.
2. Place the peppers in a food processor then pulse several times to chunk the pepper, do not liquefy.
3. Place chopped peppers into a Mason jar then cover completely with vodka.
4. Cover the jar tightly and shake jar every day for three weeks.

Dosage:

5-15 drops in water, tea, juice, or tomato juice as needed.

Notes:

Do not use this recipe if you are on ACE inhibitors.

Chamomile Tincture

Treatments:
Insomnia, colic, teething.

Ingredients:
1/2 to 1 C Dried Chamomile Flowers
1 1/2 - 1 3/4 C Boiling Water
1 1/2 - 1 3/4 C Vodka (or Rum)
Quart size glass jar with airtight lid

Instructions:
1. Fill a quart size Mason jar 1/2 to 3/4 full.
2. Pour boiling water over flowers to cover the herb.
3. Use a wooden spoon to remove gaps and air bubbles.
4. Fill the rest of the jar with vodka (or rum).
5. Tightly cover with airtight lid.
6. Store in a cool, dark place and shake daily for 4-6 weeks.
7. After 4-6 weeks, remove from cabinet, and pour through a cheesecloth-lined strainer.
8. Store in a jar or in (tincture) vials (w/ dropper).

Dosage:
Adults up to 1 teaspoon 1-3 times a day as needed.

Infants a few drops - can rub on gums or stomach for teething or colic pain.

Toddlers and older children 1/4 to 1/2 teaspoon 1-3 times daily as needed. It is especially useful for babies and young children who are having difficulty sleeping. A dose right before bedtime can help relax and sooth them for more peaceful sleep.

Echinacea Root Tincture

Ingredients:
Echinacea root
Vodka

Instructions:
1. Chop the echinacea root and add to a clean pint size glass jar.
2. Cover the root with vodka plus an extra inch.
3. Store in a cool, dark place and shake daily for 4-6 weeks.
4. After 4-6 weeks, remove from cabinet, and pour through a cheesecloth or strainer.
5. Store in a jar or in (tincture) vials (w/ dropper).

Dosage:
1/4 to 1/2 t every hour or two for adults until symptoms dissipate.

Elderberry Tincture

Treatments:
Illness, immune system boost for anyone near sickness. See Chapter 10: Additional Information, Elderberry Herb Notes / Side Effects for more information on elderberry.

Ingredients:
1 C Elderberries (Sambucus nigra)
Vodka

Instructions:
1. Place elderberries in a pint-sized Mason jar.
2. Cover elderberries with vodka leaving 1" of headspace.
3. Store in a dark place for six weeks, shake daily.
4. Strain through a fine mesh strainer into tincture bottles.
5. Store in a cool dark place.

Dosage:
Adults (12 and up): 1 t once daily for immune system boost. 1 t 3x daily when ill.
Children (5 to 12): 1/2 t once daily for immune system boost. 1/2 t 3x daily when ill.
Toddler (2 to 4): 1/8 t once daily for immune system boost. 1/8 t 3x daily when ill.

Fresh Oats Tincture

See Milky Oat Tincture.

Garlic Tincture

Treatments:
Flu/cold, contains antibacterial, antifungal, and antiviral properties. Used as an antioxidant, an immune-stimulant, anti-inflammatory, and lowers triglycerides and total cholesterol.

Ingredients:
1 C Garlic (chopped)
2 C Vodka

Instructions:
1. Chop the garlic and place in a quart-sized Mason jar.
2. Add vodka and seal.
3. Shake the jar every day for 3 weeks.
4. Strain through a fine mesh strainer.
5. Store the tincture in dark, labeled dropper bottles in a cool, dark area.

Dosage:
4-5 drops in 4 oz. of water once a day.

Notes:
[1] This tincture is not recommended for people on blood thinning medications or for people suffering from anti-coagulation disorders. [2] You may experience dizziness, nausea, and sweating after excessive intake of garlic tincture. [3] Garlic tincture may cause menstrual changes.

Ginger Rhizome Tincture

Treatments:

Nausea associated with general sickness (flu), pregnancy (morning sickness), and chemotherapy treatments. Helpful with muscle pain, soreness, arthritis, and infections.

Ingredients:

1 oz. Ginger Rhizome (root)
3 oz. Vodka (or Brandy)

Instructions:

1. Roughly chop the ginger root.
2. In a pint sized Mason jar, add the ginger and vodka (or brandy) and shake well.
3. Store in a cool, dark place for 4-6 weeks, shaking periodically.
4. Strain through cheesecloth-lined strainer and express all liquid from the mash.
5. Bottle and store in a cool, dark place.

Dosage:

Adults can handle up to three dropperfuls, three times a day. Start with a lower dose and increase as needed if symptoms don't sufficiently abate initially. Children should be started with a quarter dropperful or less and increased as needed but no more than one dropperful in a day.

Notes:

Children will generally only need one or two doses before they can discontinue.

Ginseng Root Tincture

Treatments:

Restores mental balance and well-being, cognitive function, energy, anti-inflammatory, reduce blood sugar.

Ingredients:

Hot Extraction

1 oz. (or 1/2 oz. depending on desired strength) Dried Ginseng

1 pint Boiling Water (in a non-reactive pot, do not use steel, iron, or copper)

Cold Extraction

2 oz. Dried Ginseng

1 pint Cold Water (in a non-reactive pot, do not use steel, iron, or copper)

Alcohol Extraction

3-4 oz. Dried Ginseng

8-12 oz. Vodka

8-12 oz. Distilled Water

Instructions:

Hot Extraction

1. Add one ounce of dried ginseng to a pint of boiling water in a non-metallic pot.
2. Steep this infusion for roughly 10 minutes.
3. Strain the liquid.

Cold Extraction

1. Add two ounces of dried ginseng to a pint of cold water (cold extraction requires double the ginseng as hot).
2. Steep for 8 to 12 hours.
3. Strain the liquid.

Alcohol Extraction

1. Add 3-4 ounces of dried ginseng to a mason jar.
2. Pour equal parts vodka and distilled water over the root, approximately 8-12 of each liquid.
3. Cover the ginseng completely with the alcohol and water solution.
4. Seal the jar and allow it to steep in a dark place (at room

temperature) for two weeks.
5. Strain the liquid.

Dosage:
1 teaspoon per cup of water, tea or other drink.

Notes:
Cold extractions limit the release of bitter or unpalatable elements while preserving the desirable volatile oils. Refrigerate all but the alcohol extraction. Cold and hot infusions only keep for a few days refrigerated.

Goldenseal Tincture

Treatments:
Digestion.

Ingredients:
1 T Goldenseal Leaf
1 T Orange Peel (for flavoring and some Vitamin C)
Vodka

Instructions:
1. Place each ingredient in their own jelly jar.
2. Cover each ingredient vodka (equal amount in each jar).
3. Seal and let the jars sit for one week, shaking gently once a day.
4. Strain each jar through a cheesecloth-lined strainer.
5. Combine equal parts into a tincture bottle(s).

Dosage:
2 dropperfuls in 8 oz. of water (or club soda) 15-20 minutes before a meal.

Herbal Digestion

Ingredients:
1/2 C Dried Peppermint leaves
1/4 -1/2 C Ginger Root (finely diced)
1/4 C Dried Fennel Seeds
1 1/2 C Boiling Water (approx.)
1 1/2 C Vodka or Rum (approx.)
A quart size glass jar with airtight lid

Instructions:
1. Put peppermint, ginger and fennel in glass jar and pour boiling water until they are just covered.
2. Fill the rest of the jar with vodka or rum (food grade only! no rubbing alcohol) and put on airtight lid.
3. Keep in a cool dark place for at least two weeks, but up to six, shaking daily.
4. After 2-6 weeks, strain through mesh strainer or cheesecloth and store in vials or small jars.

Dosage:
Adults 1 teaspoon (straight or in water) as needed - for heartburn indigestion or nausea, one dose usually does the trick.

Pregnant Women 1/2 teaspoon in the morning often helps with morning sickness, with additional doses if needed throughout the day.

Children 10-20 drops is usually enough or use externally.

Inflammation and Pain

Ingredients:
1/2 t Bupleurum Root Tincture
1/2 t Ginseng Root Tincture
1/2 t Licorice Root Tincture
1/2 t Echinacea Root Tincture
1/2 t Yucca Root Tincture
1/2 t Turmeric Tincture (if available)

Instructions:
1. Combine ingredients.

Dosage:
Half a dropperful a few times a day or as needed. For long-term use, consult an herbalist.

Notes:
[1] If you do not, or cannot, drink alcohol, buy/use glycerites instead of tinctures containing alcohol.

Insomnia Tincture

Treatments:
Insomnia, stress, and anxiety.

Ingredients:
3 T Dried Passionflower
3 T Dried Valerian Root
Vodka

Instructions:
1. Add the dried herbs to a jar.
2. Fill the jar with vodka.
3. Cap and shake well.
4. Store in a dark place away from sunlight and let steep for 3-5 weeks.
5. Shake occasionally.
6. Strain through a fine mesh cloth into a clean largemouth jar and squeeze out as much liquid as possible from the passionflower and valerian root.
7. Pour the liquid via funnel into tincture bottles and store in a cool, dark area.

Dosage:
10 drops per 1/4 C of water 45 minutes before bed.

Notes:
You may need to add more vodka as the herb will absorb the liquid.

Lemon Balm Leaf Tincture

Treatments:

Anxiety, stress, insomnia, depression, nervous and digestive system calming.

Ingredients:
2 C Lemon Balm Leaves
Vodka

Instructions:
1. Roughly chop the lemon balm leaves and loosely pack a pint-size mason jar.
2. Fill the jar with vodka.
3. Use a wooden spoon to push down any floaters and remove most of the bubbles.
4. Store in a cool dark place for four to six weeks, shake gently on occasion.
5. Strain through a fine mesh cloth into a clean largemouth jar and squeeze out as much liquid as possible.
6. Pour the liquid via funnel into tincture bottles and store in a cool, dark area.

Dosage:

One dropperful as needed. No need to mix in tea or dilute in water.

Notes:

Start with taking just the one dropperful to see if symptoms abate. Give the tincture at least thirty minutes to do its job before taking another dropperful.

Licorice Root Tincture

Treatments:
Aches, pains, digestion, and mood.

Ingredients:
1/2 C Dandelion Root
1/2 C Orange Peel, dried
1/2 C Yellow Dock Root
1/2 C Licorice Root
1/2 C Fennel Seed
1/4 C Burdock Root
1/4 C Calendula Flowers
1 C Water, boiling
Vodka

Instructions:
1. Roughly chop all of the herbs then combine in a quart-sized mason jar.
2. Add one-cup boiling water.
3. Stir to moisten the herbs, and then allow cooling.
4. Once cool, fill the remaining space with vodka.
5. Cover the jar and store in a cool, dark place for four to six weeks (add more vodka as necessary to keep the ingredients submerged).
6. Strain the mixture and express all stored liquid from the ingredients.
7. Pour into small brown tinctures with labels and store in a cool, dark place.

Dosage:
If being used for digestive reasons, add 12-15 dropperfuls in warm water 30 minutes before a meal.

Migraine Tincture

Treatments:
For the treatment of severe or migraine headaches.

Ingredients:
80 Proof Vodka
2 Parts Lemon Balm
1 Part Feverfew

Instructions:
1. Finely chop the fresh herbs.
2. Measure out the herbs (2 parts to 1 part) so you have enough to fill a Mason jar and leave two-inches of headspace. (Same instruction applies of using dried herbs)
3. Add the herbs to the Mason jar.
4. Add the vodka but leave enough space to shake the mixture (about 1/2 inch or so).
5. Place the lid on the jar and shake until well mixed.
6. Place in a sunny spot where it can steep for two to six weeks.
7. Shake the jar daily.
8. After steeping, strain the mixture through cheesecloth of fine strainer and discard herbs.
9. Store in tincture in dark bottles or in a cool dark place.

Dosage:
1/2 teaspoon when you feel the onset of a migraine. Repeat every 30-60 minutes until you feel the symptoms dissipate. Because of the inclusion of alcohol, ask a doctor's advice before you administer it to a child.

Notes:
The shelf life is approximately 5 years.

Milky Oat Tincture

Treatments:
Stress and nerves.

Ingredients:
1 1/2 C Milky Oats (green oats without viable seed)
Vodka

Instructions:
1. Separate the oat from the stem and pat dry as needed.
2. Place the oats and 1/2 cup of vodka in a food processor and blend to break up the oats – be careful not to over-blend and liquefy the oats.
3. Place the blended mixture in a pint-sized mason jar.
4. Add enough vodka to fill the jar.
5. Cap the jar with the lid, shake well, and store for six weeks.
6. When ready, strain tincture through a fine mesh cloth into a clean largemouth jar and squeeze out as much liquid as possible from the oats.
7. Pour the liquid via funnel into tincture bottles and store in a cool, dark area.

Dosage:
10 drops per 1/4 C of water or juice as symptoms present.

Notes:
[1] Use glycerite instead of vodka if being used as part of an alcohol cessation regimen. [2] You may need to add more vodka as the herb will absorb the liquid.

Myrrh Tincture

Treatments:
Oral care (mouthwashes and toothpastes) and sore, spongy or inflamed gums, loose teeth, Canker sores, toothache, Gingivitis, Halitosis, sore throat, or Thrush.

Ingredients:
1 part Myrrh (finely ground)
3 parts 90 Proof Alcohol (vodka does well as does brandy, scotch, and whiskey)
Mason jar with a tight-fitting lid
Coffee filter
Tincture bottle

Instructions:
1. Grind the myrrh two to three times until it is finely ground.
2. Combine 1 part ground myrrh to 3 parts alcohol in a mason jar.
3. Seal the jar tightly and shake.
4. Place the jar in a warm place out of direct sunlight.
5. Shake your jar vigorously daily for six weeks.
6. After six weeks, filter the tincture into a clean tincture bottle that has either a dropper, screw top lid, or a snug-fitting cork.
7. Allow the tincture to sit undisturbed for 2-3 days so any sediment can settle out.
8. After sedimentation, pour or syphon off the myrrh tincture and bottle it for use. It can keep for a few years in a cool dark place.

Dosage:
When issues arise, dissolve 1/4-1/2 teaspoon sea salt in a cup of warm water then add 1-teaspoon myrrh tincture. Swish the mixture in your mouth for 2-3 minutes then spit out. Repeat multiple times daily.
For preventative use, use once daily.

Nerve Pain

Ingredients:
1 t St. John's Wort Tincture
1 t Skullcap Tincture
1 t Fresh Oats Tincture
1t Licorice Root Tincture
1/2 dropper-full Ginger Rhizome Tincture
1/2 dropper-full Blue Vervain Tincture

Instructions:
1. Combine ingredients.

Dosage:
1 dropperful every half hour or as needed during an emergency. For chronic pain, 2 to 4 dropperfuls a day.

Passionflower Tincture

Treatments:
Calm anxiety, reduce muscle tension, and improve sleep by regulating melatonin.

Ingredients:
Vodka
Passionflower, dried or fresh*
Distilled Water (for fresh passionflower)

* If using fresh passionflower, harvest at the early flowering stage for greater potency. Don't use just the flower though. Use the flower, leaves, and vine/stem.

Instructions (dried passionflower):
1. Fill a pint size Mason jar half full of dried passionflower.
2. Fill jar with vodka then seal.
3. Shake vigorously once a day for 4 weeks.
4. Strain out the herb using a funnel and an unbleached coffee filter into tincture bottles.
5. Label and store in a cool and dark place.

Instructions (fresh passionflower):
1. Roughly chop plant parts, weigh, and add to a blender.
2. Add 3oz. vodka and 1 oz. distilled water for every 2 oz. of passionflower.
3. Blend until well combined (2-4 quick presses of the button).
4. Pour mixture into pint size Mason jar and seal.
5. Shake mixture daily for two weeks.
6. Strain out the herb using a funnel and an unbleached coffee filter into tincture bottles.
7. Label and store in a cool and dark place.

Dosage:
Take 1-2 dropperfuls in a small amount of water 3-5 daily, or as needed.

Shepherd's Purse Tincture

Treatments:
Bleeding from nose bleeds, menstruation, and childbirth (during and postpartum).

Ingredients:
Shepherd's Purse
Vodka (or brandy)

Instructions:
1. Fill a mason jar 3/4 full with freshly harvested Shepherd's Purse.
2. Pour vodka, or brandy, over the herb, up to 1/2 inch from the top of the jar, making sure to cover the herb completely.
3. Shake once a day for a week and then set aside in a dark spot for three more weeks.
4. Strain the material in a cheesecloth lined strainer and squeeze out any additional liquid.
5. Transfer to tincture bottle and store in cool dark place.

Dosage:
10-20 drops by mouth as needed.

Skullcap Tincture

Treatments:

Insomnia, anxiety, stroke, and paralysis caused by stroke. Can also be used for fever, high cholesterol, hardening of the arteries (atherosclerosis), rabies, epilepsy, nervous tension, allergies, skin infections, inflammation, and spasms.

Ingredients:

Skullcap leaves
Vodka

Instructions:

1. Fill the jar 1/2 full with dried skullcap leaves.
2. Pour vodka over the leaves until the jar is full.
3. Use a wooden spoon to remove gaps and air bubbles.
4. Store out of direct sunlight for 4-6 weeks.
5. Open and stir daily the first week then allow it to sit for an additional 4-5 weeks, shaking once or twice a week.
6. To strain, line a strainer with cheesecloth and pour mixture over. Squeeze out any liquid from the skullcap before composting.
7. Bottle in tincture bottles and store in a cool, dark place.

Dosage:

One dropperful as needed.

St. John's Wort Tincture

Treatments:

Depression, nervous tension, stress, and overall mood. Also used for menopausal symptoms, attention-deficit hyperactivity disorder (ADHD), and obsessive-compulsive disorder (OCD).

Ingredients:

Vodka

Fresh St. John's Wort (aerial part of the plant, meaning parts of the plant completely exposed to air)

Instructions:

1. Collect enough plant material to fill a sterilized glass jar halfway.
2. Fill jar with vodka.
3. Shake the mixture daily for 4 weeks.
4. Strain out the herb using fine mesh cheesecloth then bottle via funnel into tincture bottles.
5. Label and store in a cool and dark place.

Dosage:

Take 15-20 drops of tincture three times a day.

Notes:

[1] Use glycerite instead of vodka if being used as part of an alcohol cessation regimen. [2] You may need to add more vodka as the herb will absorb the liquid.

Tincture of Yarrow

Treatments:

Relieves fever, shortens duration of colds and flus, improves relaxation during illness, and relieves cramps. Can also be used on cuts, scrapes, bites, punctures.

Ingredients:

Yarrow Flowers
Vodka

Instructions:

1. Harvest enough Yarrow flowers to fill one and a half pint size mason jars.
2. Cut the wilted yarrow into small pieces using a sharp kitchen knife or scissors and re-fill one of the jars (once cut up, you should have enough to fill the jar leaving about 1" to 1/2" of 'headspace'.)
3. Cover the plant material with vodka making sure all of the yarrow is submerged.
4. Cap and store in a cool, dark place for six weeks, shaking daily.
5. After six weeks, strain the plant material from the liquid.
6. Bottle in a clean dropper bottle and label.

Dosage:

For fever, colds and flus (illness), and cramps, place 1/2 to 1 dropperful of tincture under the tongue 3 times daily. For acute conditions, take smaller and/or more frequent doses, such as 1/4 teaspoon (1/2 dropperful) every hour.

For cuts, scrapes, bites, and punctures, dilute the tincture in water and soak a cotton cloth then place the cloth over the affected area.

Notes:

For an alcohol free tincture, use boiling water (1/4 jar) and glycerite (remaining space ~3/4 jar). See *Yarrow Skin Wash* in Chapter 8: Salves.

Thyme Tincture

Treatments:
Acne, antiseptic and antifungal properties.

Ingredients:
Thyme
Vodka

Instructions:
1. Fill up glass jar (Mason) with herb halfway.
2. Add vodka so that level of the liquid is at least two inches above the herb.
3. Seal jar tightly.
4. Label jar with date.
5. Shake two times per day for one month.
6. Filter liquid into tincture bottles while expressing liquid from the thyme.

Dosage:
For acne, dilute the tincture in water and soak a cotton cloth then place the cloth over the affected area like a facial mask for five minutes.
For antifungal issues like athletes foot, use full strength 1/2 dropperful at a time between toes or on nail bed twice daily.

Turmeric Tincture

Treatments:

Inflammation and general heart health (regulates blood pressure and reduces the risk of blood clots). Also functions as a blood thinner.

Ingredients:
Turmeric Root
Vodka

Instructions:
1. Roughly chop the turmeric root.
2. In a pint sized Mason jar, add the turmeric and vodka and shake well.
3. Store in a cool, dark place for 4-6 weeks, shaking periodically.
4. Strain through cheesecloth-lined strainer and express all liquid from the mash.
5. Bottle and store in a cool, dark place.

Dosage:
1 dropperful three times a day.

Notes:

[1] Pregnant women should avoid this tincture and any other combination of tinctures or supplements containing high doses of turmeric due to its blood thinning properties. [2] Wear gloves and an apron when chopping turmeric as the root will stain the hands and clothing. Hands stains will remain for several days.

Valerian Root Tincture

Treatments:
Stress and anxiety.

Ingredients:
1 part Dried Valerian Root
2 parts Vodka

Instructions:
1. Fill the jar halfway with valerian root.
2. Fill the jar with vodka.
3. Cap and shake well.
4. Store in a dark place away from sunlight and let steep for 3-5 weeks.
5. Shake occasionally.
6. Strain through a fine mesh cloth into a clean largemouth jar and squeeze out as much liquid as possible.
7. Pour the liquid via funnel into tincture bottles and store in a cool, dark area.

Dosage:
10 drops per 1/4 C of water or juice as symptoms present.

Notes:
[1] Use glycerite instead of vodka if being used as part of an alcohol cessation regimen. [2] You may need to add more vodka as the herb will absorb the liquid.

Yucca Root Tincture

Treatments:

Compromised immune systems, root is high in vitamin C and antioxidants so it stimulates the production of white blood cells to fight infections and viruses.

Ingredients:
Yucca Root
Vodka

Instructions:
1. Cut up the yucca root and fill a pint sized Mason jar halfway.
2. Cover the yucca root by at least one inch with vodka.
3. Cap and shake well.
4. Store in a dark place away from sunlight and let steep for 4-6 weeks.
5. Shake occasionally.
6. Strain through a fine mesh cloth into a clean largemouth jar and squeeze out as much liquid as possible.
7. Pour the liquid via funnel into tincture bottles and store in a cool, dark area.

Dosage:
3-5 milliliters in tea or water 2-3 times a day.

Chapter 10 – Additional Information

In addition to the recipes contained herein, I was also presented with a wealth of information on a variety of topics. The information is worth noting so I decided to include it here in an 'Additional Information' chapter.

> Please note that neither the author nor the publisher endorses or assumes any liability for the following information or for any of the proposed treatments. You are instructed to discuss all medical matters with your preferred healthcare provider prior to incorporating any of the following into your diet or lifestyle.

The information presented in Chapter 10 has been cleaned up with headings and text inserts for readability.

Cayenne: A Remarkable Healing Herb

The following text associated with the healthful uses of cayenne is attributed to Dr. Roopa Chari in its entirety. Every effort was made to verify the contents due to the original source material being cobbled together from a variety of resources by others. For more information on Dr. Roopa Chari, her practice, or for contact information, please visit her medical offices website. She and her husband are located in Encinitas, California.

* * *

Cayenne is a gift to humanity because it has more health benefits than any other food or herb on earth. There are over 3000 scientific studies listed in the National Library of Medicine to support the use of cayenne in preventing and reversing many common health ailments. It is miraculous that a simple fruit like cayenne has healing benefits for a wide assortment of ailments. It has been used as a food, a spice, and an herbal medicine for over 9000 years.

All hot peppers are botanically called capsicum. They are put into different groups depending on the various species, such as capsicum annum and capsicum frutescens. Cayenne refers to one variety of capsicum, but over the years it has become synonymous with capsicum and refers to most hot varieties of chilies.

The potency of cayenne is determined by the intensity of its heat. This is determined by the quantity of the chemicals in cayenne and its resins. The more of these chemicals that are in cayenne and the hotter it is the stronger it is indicates it is more effective in healing. The heat is measured in heat units, which are called Scoville Units or heat units.

Capsicum is rated between 0 to 300,000 heat units. Most cayenne peppers are between 30,000 to 80,000 heat units. Paprika has no heat and is rated 0 heat units. Jalapeno peppers are between 50,000 to 80,000 heat units, Serrano peppers are approximately 100,000 heat units, African Bird Peppers are 200,000 heat units and Mexican habaneros are between 250,000-300,000 heat units.

A fresh cayenne chili pepper is nutrient rich and contains:

- Water
- Carbohydrate
- Starch
- Protein
- Fiber
- Vitamin C
- Capsaicinoids
- Beta Carotene
- Iron
- Phosphorus
- Calcium

Chili Peppers are also low in fat and contain the right kind of fat: 66% of the fat as linoleic and 5% as linolenic acid which are two essential fats in the diet of humans.

The variety of colors found in chili peppers contain thousands of bioflavinoids and carotenoids which may be responsible for the healing properties of cayenne and they heal heart cells and protect your heart.

There are vitamins in cayenne that will destroy bacteria and enhance your immune system. There is also no other herb that will increase your blood flow faster than cayenne.

According to Dr. Richard Schulze, an internationally recognized herbalist, "there is no other herb stronger or more effective than cayenne to make immediate physiological and metabolic changes in the body."

Capsaicin, has been proven to protect your DNA and cells from attack by toxic molecules such as from tobacco, and other toxins. They can also prevent cancer by inhibiting the transformation of cells, which eventually form cancer.

The following are just some of the conditions which cayenne may be used to treat:

- Allergies
- Arthritis
- Asthma
- Blood circulation problems
- Cancer prevention
- Colds and flus
- Congestive heart failure
- Constipation
- Diabetes
- Heart disease
- Hemorrhoids
- High blood pressure
- High cholesterol
- Obesity
- Osteoarthritis
- Stops bleeding (internally or externally)
- Stroke

However, it is not just a matter of using Cayenne. The quality of the cayenne is extremely important. You should keep a bottle of this cayenne tincture or bag the cayenne powder in your kitchen, place some in the glove compartment of your cars, etc. as it can be life saving!

Specific remedies using Cayenne include:

- For Health Maintenance: Put 5 drops in water or juice and drink it 1-3 times a day. You can slowly increase the dosage.
- For a bleeding wound: Liberally flush the wound with cayenne tincture or pack with cayenne powder and apply pressure to the wound.
- Depending on the severity of the bleeding, also take 1-10 full dropper of the tincture in a few ounces of water in your mouth. Or just put directly into your mouth.

Attributed to Dr. Roopa Chari, M.D.

Cinnamon and Honey

As I began forming the outline and conducting research for this book, I was presented with the following excerpt by the administrator of a trusted online forum. According to the admin, the author and their family have been making homemade natural remedies in a remote location for many generations. Unfortunately, the author(s) have chosen to remain anonymous.

* * *

I was talking to some people at church about this [cinnamon and honey] then, low and behold, I found this.

Honey is the only food on the planet that will not spoil or rot. What it will do is what some call 'turning to sugar'. In reality, honey is always honey. However, when left in a cool dark place for a long time it will 'crystallize'. When this happens, loosen the lid, boil some water and sit the honey container in the hot water, but turn off the heat and let it liquefy naturally. It is then as good as it ever was. Never boil honey or put it in a microwave. This will kill the enzymes in the honey.

Bet the drug companies won't like this one getting around. Facts on honey and cinnamon: It is found that a mixture of honey and cinnamon cures most diseases. Honey is produced in most of the countries of the world. Scientists of today also accept honey as a 'Ram Ban' (very effective) medicine for all kinds of diseases. Honey can be used without side effects for many kinds of diseases.

Today's science says that even though honey is sweet, when it is taken in the right dosage as a medicine, it does not harm even diabetic patients. [The following was] Researched by western scientists:

Arthritis

Arthritis patients may take daily (morning and night) one cup of hot water with two tablespoons of honey and one small teaspoon of cinnamon powder. When taken regularly even chronic arthritis can be cured. In a recent research conducted at the Copenhagen University, it was found that when the doctors treated their patients with a mixture of one tablespoon honey and half teaspoon cinnamon powder before breakfast, they found that within a week (out of the 200 people so treated) practically 73 patients [36.5%] were totally relieved of pain.

Within a month, most all the patients who could not walk or move around because of arthritis now started walking without pain.

Bad Breath

People of South America, gargle with one teaspoon of honey and cinnamon powder mixed in hot water first thing in the morning so their breath stays fresh throughout the day.

Bladder Infections

Take two tablespoons of cinnamon powder and one teaspoon of honey in a glass of lukewarm water and drink it. It destroys the germs in the bladder.

Cancer

Recent research in Japan and Australia has revealed that advanced cancer of the stomach and bones have been cured successfully. Patients suffering from these kinds of cancer should daily take one tablespoon of honey with one teaspoon of cinnamon powder three times a day for one month.

Cholesterol

Two tablespoons of honey and three teaspoons of cinnamon powder mixed in 16 ounces of tea water given to a cholesterol patient was found to reduce the level of bad cholesterol in the blood by 10 percent within two hours. As mentioned for arthritic patients, when taken three times a day, any chronic cholesterol is cured. According to information received in the same Journal, pure honey taken with food daily relieves complaints of cholesterol as well.

Colds

Those suffering from common or severe colds should take one tablespoon lukewarm honey with 1/4 spoon cinnamon powder daily for three days. This process will cure most chronic cough, cold, and, clear the sinuses.

Fatigue

Recent studies have shown that the sugar content of honey is more helpful rather than being detrimental to the strength of the body. Senior citizens who take honey and cinnamon powder in equal parts are more alert and flexible. Dr. Milton, who has done research, says that a half tablespoon of honey taken in a glass of water and sprinkled with cinnamon powder, even when the vitality of the body starts to decrease, when taken daily after brushing and in the afternoon at about 3:00 P.M., the vitality of the body increases within a week.

Gas

According to the studies done in India and Japan, it is revealed that when honey is taken with cinnamon powder the stomach is relieved of gas.

Hearing Loss

Daily morning and night honey and cinnamon powder, taken in equal parts helps alleviate hearing issues [associated with ringing cloudiness resulting from association with prolonged high decibel activities. This treatment does NOT restore lost hearing (deafness).]

Heart Disease

Make a paste of honey and cinnamon powder, apply it on bread instead of jelly and jam, and eat it regularly for breakfast. It reduces the cholesterol in the arteries and saves the patient from heart attack. Also, those who have already had an attack, when they do this process daily, they are kept miles away from the next attack. Regular use of the above process relieves loss of breath and strengthens the heartbeat. In America and Canada, various nursing homes have treated patients successfully and have found that as one ages the arteries and veins lose their flexibility and become clogged; honey and cinnamon revitalizes the arteries and the veins.

Immune System

Daily use of honey and cinnamon powder strengthens the immune system and protects the body from bacterial and viral attacks. Scientists have found that honey has various vitamins and iron in large amounts. Constant use of honey strengthens the white blood corpuscles (where DNA is contained) to fight bacterial and viral diseases.

Indigestion

Cinnamon powder sprinkled on two tablespoons of honey taken before food is eaten relieves acidity and digests the heaviest of meals

Influenza

A scientist in Spain has proved that honey contains a natural 'Ingredient' that kills the influenza germs and saves the patient from flu. [May also aid in preventing and/or shortening of Corona Virus symptoms.]

Longevity

Tea made with honey and cinnamon powder, when taken regularly, arrests the ravages of old age. Use four teaspoons of honey, one teaspoon of cinnamon powder, and three cups of boiling water to make a tea. Drink 1/4 cup, three to four times a day. It keeps the skin fresh and soft and arrests old age. Life spans increase and even a 100 year old will start performing the chores of a 20-year-old.

Pimples

Three tablespoons of honey and one teaspoon of cinnamon powder paste. Apply this paste on the pimples (acne) before sleeping and wash it off the next morning with warm water. When done daily for two weeks, it removes all pimples from the root.

Raspy or Sore Throat

When throat has a tickle or is raspy, take one tablespoon of honey, and sip until gone. Repeat every three hours until throat is without symptoms.

Skin Infections

Applying honey and cinnamon powder in equal parts on the affected parts cures eczema, ringworm and all types of skin infections.

Upset Stomach

Honey taken with cinnamon powder cures stomachache and clears stomach ulcers from its root.

Weight Loss

Daily in the morning one half hour before breakfast and on an empty stomach, and at night before sleeping, add 2 tablespoons honey and 1/4-1/2 teaspoon of cinnamon powder to a boiled cup of water. When taken regularly, it reduces the weight of even the most obese person. In addition, drinking this mixture regularly does not allow the fat to accumulate in the body even though the person may eat a high calorie diet.

Elderberry Herb Notes / Side Effects

Elderberry, as an ingredient, seems to be surrounded by myth, fear, legend, and providence. Knowing that, I was fortunate that a contributor provided the following information regarding Elderberry.

* * *

Latin Name: Sambucus nigra

Common Names: Elder, Elderberry, Black Elder, European Elder, European Elderberry, European Black Elferberry, and North American Elderberry

Properties: Antioxidant, diaphoretic, diuretic, laxative, immune-boosting, anti-inflammatory

Treatments: Immune system boost, coughs, colds, flu, bacterial infections, viral infections, tonsillitis, lower cholesterol, improved vision and heart health.

Indicated For: Cancer, HIV, asthma and bronchitis, reduce inflammation of the urinary tract and bladder. Infusions of the fruit are said to be beneficial for nerve disorders, back pain, and have been used to reduce inflammation of the urinary tract and bladder.

Are Elderberries Poisonous? Most species of Sabcucus berries are edible when picked ripe and then cooked. Both the skin and pulp can be eaten. However, it is important to note that most uncooked berries and other parts of plants from this genus are poisonous. Sambucus nigra is the variety of Elderberry that is most often used for health benefits as it is the only variety considered to be non-toxic even when not cooked, but it is still recommended to cook the berries at least a little to enhance their taste and digestibility.

There is also an excellent article on the Organic Prepper website *Elderberry Extract for the Flu: Nature's "Tamiflu."* [Full URL: https://www.theorganicprepper.com/elderberry-extract-natures-tamiflu/]. I used the Elderberry Extract that I got from Walgreens with very good results during the Mexican flu epidemic - I'm one of those that don't get the flu shot.

God's RX

Lastly, the same family that provided the information on Cinnamon and Honey also provided the following information regarding God's earthly medicine cabinet and the clues/resemblances left behind to guide us in our healing.

* * *

I am sure we have all seen this but it worth repeating.

It's been said that God first separated the salt water from the fresh, made dry land, planted a garden, made animals and fish. [He did] all [of this] before making a human. He made and provided what we'd need before we were born. These [fruits, nuts, and vegetables] are best and more powerful when eaten raw. We're such slow learners.

God left us great clues as to what foods help what part of our body!

God's Pharmacy! Amazing!

Avocadoes, Eggplant, Pears

Avocadoes, Eggplant, and Pears target the health and function of the womb and cervix of the female. [They also] look just like these organs. Today's research shows that when a woman eats one avocado a week, it balances hormones, sheds unwanted birth weight, and prevents cervical cancers. It takes exactly nine months to grow an avocado from blossom to ripened fruit. How profound is this?

There are over 14,000 photolytic chemical constituents of nutrition in each one of these foods. Modern science has only studied and named about 150 of them.

Carrots

A sliced carrot looks like the human eye. The pupil, iris, and radiating lines look just like the human eye. [Modern] science now shows carrots greatly enhance blood flow to and function of the eyes.

Celery, Bok Choy, Rhubarb

Celery, Bok Choy, Rhubarb, and many more look just like bones and specifically target bone strength. Bones are 23% sodium and these foods are 23% sodium. If you don't have enough sodium in your diet, the body pulls it from the bones, thus making them weak. These foods replenish the skeletal needs of the body.

Figs

Figs are full of seeds and hang in twos when they grow. Figs increase the mobility of male sperm and increase the numbers of sperm as well to help overcome male sterility.

Grapes

Grapes hang in a cluster that has the shape of the heart. Each grape looks like a blood cell and all of the research today shows grapes are also a profound heart and blood revitalizing food.

Kidney Beans

Kidney Beans actually heal and help maintain kidney function and yes, they look exactly like the human kidneys.

Olives

Olives assist the health and function of the ovaries

Onions

Onions look like the body's cells. Today's research shows onions help clear waste materials from all of the body cells. They even produce tears which wash the epithelial layers of the eyes. A working companion, Garlic, also helps eliminate waste materials and dangerous free radicals from the body.

Oranges

Oranges, Grapefruits, and other Citrus fruits look just like the mammary glands of the female and actually assist the health of the breasts and the movement of lymph in and out of the breasts.

Sweet Potatoes

Sweet Potatoes look like the pancreas and actually balance the glycemic index of diabetics.

Tomatoes

A tomato has four chambers and is red. The heart has four chambers and is red. Research shows that tomatoes are loaded with lycopene and are indeed pure heart and blood food.

Walnuts

A walnut looks like a little brain, a left and right hemisphere, upper cerebrums, and lower cerebellums. Even the wrinkles or folds on the nut are just like the neo-cortex. We now know [that] walnuts help develop more than three dozen neuron-transmitters for brain function.

Kidney Stones

There are several herbs, or combinations of herbs, that can help with different aspects of kidney stones. The following is a brief list of herbal remedies for dissolving, preventing, and addressing kidney stones.

* * *

Aloe

Aloe can be taken internally in the form of pure aloe juice. Take 1/4 C daily for no more than 2 weeks at a time. Aloe contains acemannan, which slows the rate of crystal formation.

Basil Juice and Honey

A mixture of 1 t basil juice and honey may be taken daily to strengthen kidney function and check stone formation.

Birch Leaf

The birch leaf stimulates urination and stops spasms. It also can be ingested in the form of tea in the amount of 1 C three times a day.

Black Cherry Juice

Black cherry juice lowers uric acid levels and checks stone formation.

Chanca Piedra

Chanca piedra is an herb that is taken internally in the tincture from, which dissolves calcium stones.

Cramp Bark

Cramp bark extracts reduces pain and muscle spasm due to stones.

Cranberry

Cranberries help in dissolving stones from the kidney.

Dandelion Root and Fennel Seeds

A combination of dandelion root extracts and fennel seeds can easily flush out kidney stones.

Gravel Root

Gravel root is effective in helping one getting rid of this problem.

Goldenrod

Goldenrod herb cleanses urinary tract of stones.

Joe Pye Weed, Meadowsweet, Sarsaparilla

Herbs like joe-pye weed, meadowsweet, and sarsaparilla may be used in the form of tea to remove kidney stones naturally.

Juniper Berry and Marshmallow Root

Juniper berries and marshmallow root also break down kidney stones in to tiny pieces and enable easy flushing out.

Khella

Khella is an herbal remedy that helps the urinary tract heal after a stone passes. It can be taken in a variety of forms in the amount of 20 mg daily.

Kid Clear

Herbal supplements such as Kid Clear capsules are also highly beneficial in dissolving kidney stones naturally without any side effects.

Lemon Juice and Hydrangea

A combination of lemon juice and hydrangea herb extracts reduces stone size and helps in eliminating them.

Lime, Cayenne, Maple Syrup

Every morning, drink a mixture of 8 oz. distilled water, the juice of one lime, 15 drops of hot cayenne extract, and maple syrup for taste. This drink dissolves stones from the kidney magically.

Marshmallow Root

Marshmallow root helps cleanse the kidneys and expel kidney stones. It can also be taken as tea in the amount of 1 quart daily.

Nettles, Horsetails, St John's Wort

Nettles, horsetails, and St John's Wort prevent bleeding due to stones.

Varuna

Varuna blocks an enzyme that is necessary for the formation of calcium oxalate stones. It comes in the form of a loose tea, and can be prepared by steeping 1 T in 1 C of water. Drink three times a day.

Yarrow Leaf, Wild Yam Root, Corn Silk

Yarrow leaf, wild yam root, corn silk may be used as tea. These herbs are effective in dissolving stones from the kidney. See Chapter 5: General Home Remedies, Kidney Stone Tea for additional ingredients when making a tea.

Thank you for purchasing and reading through the recipes and information contained in *Home Remedies, Poultices, Salves, & Tinctures*. I hope you will consider visiting the Amazon website to leave a review so others may know what you thought of the information.

Other books by David J. Kershner:

Non-Fiction

Preparing to Prepare: A General Guide to Self-Sufficiency & Preparedness

Just a Small Gathering, Volume 1: A Guide to Entertaining Small Groups of Family and Friends

Fiction

Foreign & Domestic, Part I – When Rome Stumbles

Foreign & Domestic, Part II – Hannibal is at the Gates

Foreign & Domestic, Part III – By the Dawn's Early Light

Foreign & Domestic, Part IV – Colder Weather

Foreign & Domestic, Part V – A Time for Reckoning

Index